FLUID AND ELECTROLYTE DISORDERS

Edited by **Usman Mahmood**

Fluid and Electrolyte Disorders
http://dx.doi.org/10.5772/intechopen.72967
Edited by Usman Mahmood

Contributors

Mireia Martínez Cortés, Pedro Gurillo Muñoz, John Andrew Sayer, Holly Mabillard, Gilda Diaz-Fuentes, Sindhaghatta Venkatram, Bharat Bajantri, Vanessa Heron, Caius Breazu, Adrian Bartos, Dana Monica Bartos, Vinay Srinivasa

First published in London, United Kingdom, 2019 by IntechOpen
IntechOpen is the global imprint of INTECHOPEN LIMITED, registered in England and Wales, registration number: 11086078, The Shard, 25th floor, 32 London Bridge Street
London, SE19SG – United Kingdom
Printed in Croatia

British Library Cataloguing-in-Publication Data
A catalogue record for this book is available from the British Library

Additional hard and PDF copies can be obtained from orders@intechopen.com

Fluid and Electrolyte Disorders, Edited by Usman Mahmood
p. cm.
Print ISBN 978-1-78923-921-8
Online ISBN 978-1-78923-922-5
eBook (PDF) ISBN 978-1-83881-181-5

For EU product safety concerns:
IN TECH d.o.o., Prolaz Marije Krucifikse Kozulić 3, 51000 Rijeka, Croatia,
info@intechopen.com or visit our website at intechopen.com.

Meet the editor

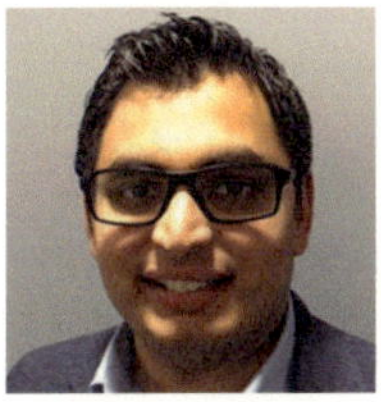

Usman Mahmood is a consultant nephrologist at Darling Downs Hospital and Health Service, Australia. He underwent postgraduate training in various public hospitals across three different states and has a range of experience in various areas of nephrology and general medicine, including both metropolitan and indigenous healthcare. His special interests include: chronic kidney disease, fluid and electrolyte disorders, renal vasculitides, hemodialysis, general medical conditions, hypertension management, lupus nephritis, glomerulonephritis, and kidney transplantation. He has authored a number of book chapters and has published in various peer-reviewed journals. Dr. Mahmood also enjoys teaching junior medical staff, including medical students. He can speak four languages and is well equipped to look after patients from a subcontinent background.

Contents

Preface

Welcome to *Fluid and Electrolyte Disorders*. This book is intended to offer an up-to-date clinical text for medical residents, fellows, practicing physicians, and nephrologists in a simple and easy-to-understand format. Fluid and electrolyte disorders are frequently encountered in clinical practice. Our understanding of the physiology and biochemistry of these disorders has greatly expanded in recent years. This book aims to discuss the current evidence regarding the physiology, basic fundamentals, clinical presentation, and management of these disorders and will help clinicians to manage these disorders effectively. It also aims to bridge the gap between pathophysiology and clinical manifestation of these disorders. All chapters have been extensively revised and bound to include the latest developments in the field.

I would like to acknowledge the support of Ms. Marijana Francetic throughout the process of publication, and would like to dedicate this book to my father, M.A. Nasir, and my late mother who helped me at every step of my life.

I hope readers will find this open-access text a valuable educational resource.

Usman Mahmood
Darling Downs Hospital and Health Service
Queensland, Australia

Chapter 1

Fluids and Sodium Imbalance: Clinical Implications

Gilda Diaz-Fuentes, Bharat Bajantri and
Sindhaghatta Venkatram

Additional information is available at the end of the chapter

http://dx.doi.org/10.5772/intechopen.79121

Abstract

Fluids and electrolytes are basic components of the human body and essential for the survival of most species. Any imbalance can potentially lead to serious conditions and death. The replacement of fluids and electrolytes has been used since the ancient age. Modern medicine still requires certain degree of expertise in these areas, which ranges from simple replacement in patients with mild illness to a more complex management in critically ill or hospitalized patients. Training and education in the evaluation and management of patients with fluids and electrolyte abnormalities are fundamental for patient's outcomes. Severe sodium abnormalities are associated with increased morbidity and mortality, and they are markers of poor outcomes. This review presents a concise discussion of frequently asked questions in the evaluation and management of patients with fluids and sodium abnormalities.

Keywords: hypernatremia, hyponatremia, fluids, normal saline, ringer lactate, albumin

1. Introduction

The serum sodium (sNa) concentration and thus serum osmolality (sOsm) are closely controlled by water homeostasis, which is mediated by thirst, arginine vasopressin, and the kidneys. A disruption in this delicate balance is manifested as an abnormality in the sNa concentration—hyponatremia or hypernatremia and/or hemodynamic instability.

Fluid administration is an integral part of the clinician's armamentarium to manage a wide variety of clinical conditions, which range from mild dehydration to more life-threatening conditions like shock or trauma.

The goal of this review is to provide a concise discussion regarding fluids and sodium imbalance with an attempt to answer practical clinical questions on those areas. We focus in discussing basics physiological principles, and addressing the most common clinical challenges encountered by the practicing clinician.

1.1. Basic physiologic principle of fluids and sodium

The human body is composed of approximately 60% of water of which two-third are in the intracellular space and one-third in the extracellular space. The extracellular space is composed by the intravascular compartment (~8%), the interstitial compartment (~25%) and the transcellular compartment like cerebrospinal, pericardial fluid, which is very small [1, 2]. In the healthy individual, the extracellular fluid (ECF) and intracellular fluid (ICF) are in osmotic equilibrium, water moves from areas of greater solute concentration to establish equilibrium. Additionally, osmotically active substance shifts water from lower osmolarity to higher osmolarity areas. This is an important concept to understand when we administer intravenous fluids (IVF), as the distribution of fluids is based on the type of fluid administered.

There is a delicate and complicated transport system of water through cell membranes to maintain fluids and electrolyte balance. Sodium is the predominant cation in the extracellular compartment, which is electro-neutralized by chloride (Cl) and bicarbonate (HCO_3) as anions. In the intracellular space, potassium (K) is the major intracellular cation that is neutralized by many organic and nonorganic anions. The differential distribution of Na and K is tightly regulated by the sodium pump (Na-K ATPase) [1, 2]. Most osmotically active Na and K are dissolved and are sourced mostly from food intake. The body's ability to store sodium in tissues (bone, cartilage, connective tissue, etc.) prevents large fluctuations in the sNa levels despite erratic sodium intake [3, 4]. Most of the components in the intracellular compartment are too large to be able to cross membranes exerting little osmotic pressure.

Estimating the ECF volume based on sNa is highly prone to errors in clinical judgment. The volume in both, intracellular and extracellular fluids is primarily determined by the concentration of effective solutes that attract water by osmosis. Sodium and its attendant monovalent anions are the most prevalent effective solutes in ECF volume. The concentration of Na is determined by content of Na as well as volume of water. The primary tonicity receptor is located in the hypothalamic osmoreceptor, which is in charge to regulate the antidiuretic hormone (ADH) or vasopressin. The absence of ADH prevents aquaporin insertion on the luminal surfaces of collecting ducts in the nephrons forming hypotonic urine. The osmoreceptor is linked to both the thirst center and the vasopressin release center via nerve connections. There is a genetic susceptibility to hyponatremia linked to the gene coding for TRPV4 [2, 5–8]. Disease states releasing ectopic vasopressin or affecting vasopressin receptors will present with hyponatremia. Less prominent but important trigger for the regulation of vasopressin is large changes in effective arterial blood volume and blood pressure. Baroreceptors or stretch receptors in the carotid sinus and aortic arch are surrogates that detect changes in effective arterial blood volume. Nausea, pain, stress, and a number of other stimuli, including some drugs can also cause release of vasopressin [5].

http://dx.doi.org/10.5772/intechopen.79121

2. Fluids

Intravenous fluids are one of the commonest used medications in hospitalized patients. They can be broadly categorized as crystalloids and colloids. Crystalloid solutions contain water, electrolytes with or without glucose. Colloids solutions contain albumin, starch, or other blood products. Fluids can be isotonic, hypotonic, or hypertonic.

Crystalloids: Common crystalloid solutions include 0.9%-normal saline (NS), 0.45%NS, lactated Ringers solutions (LR), Plasma-Lyte, and dextrose in water. Solutions with electrolyte compositions closer to that of plasma are called balanced fluids. Composition of commonly used crystalloids can be seen in **Table 1**.

Colloids: They can be divided into natural or synthetic. Natural colloidal solutions include red blood cells, fresh frozen plasma, and human albumin. Indications for the use of packed red cell and fresh frozen plasma are specific; they provide oxygen carrying capacity and clotting factors, respectively. Discussion regarding the use of red blood cells and plasma is beyond the scope of this review.

Synthetic colloidal solutions include hetastarch and dextran. They are used for volume expansion and include hetastarch and dextran.

Colloids can be categorized as hypo oncotic (e.g., gelatins, 4 or 5% albumin) and hyper oncotic (e.g., dextrans, hydroxyethyl starches (HES), and 20 or 25% albumin) solutions. **Table 2** describes the composition of commonly used colloids.

Indications for the use of either crystalloids or colloids depend of the clinical condition. Volume expansion by fluids is dependent on their osmolality and oncotic pressure. Isotonic fluids will distribute equally to all fluid compartments without a significant shift across

Solution	Na+ (mEq/L)	Cl− (mEq/L)	K+ (mEq/L)	Ca++ (mEq/L)	Lactate (mEq/L)	Glucose (g/l)	pH	Osmolarity (mOsm/L)
0.9%NS	154	154	0	0	0	0	pH 5.6 (4.5–7.0)	308
0.45 saline (1/2 saline)	77	77	0	0	0	0	5.0 (4.5–7)	154
3% saline	513	513	0	0	0	0	5.0 (4.5–7)	1026
Ringers lactate	130	109	4	3	28	0	6.5	272
Plasma-Lyte A*	140	98	5	0	8	0	7.4	294
5% dextrose	0	0	0	0	0	50	5.0	260

*Also contains magnesium 3 mEq/L, acetate 27 mEq/L, gluconate 23 mEq/L.

Table 1. Composition of crystalloids.

Fluid	Na+ (mEq/L)	Cl− (mEq/L)	Colloidal oncotic pressure (mm Hg)	Osmolarity (mOsm/L)
Albumin 5%	130–160	130–160	20	308
Albumin 25%	154	154	100	308
Hetastarch (6%)-NaCl	154	154	30	310
Gelatins (gelofusine 4%)	154	154	33	310
Dextran 70 + NaCl	154	154	60	310

Table 2. Composition of colloids.

cellular or vascular planes. However, hypertonic solutions will move fluids from intracellular and interstitial space into the intravascular compartment, while hypotonic fluids will result in shift of fluids from intravascular space to interstitial and intracellular compartments. Volume expansion of the intravascular compartment with colloids depends on the oncotic pressure.

The most common clinical indications for fluid administration are:

- Replacement of volume losses
- Maintenance of fluids and electrolyte balance
- Correction of electrolyte or acid-base disorders
- Persistent hypoglycemia or hyperglycemia
- Provision of a source of fuel (glucose)
- Intravenous administration of medication.

2.1. Question 1: which fluids are more effective—colloids or crystalloids?

Fluid resuscitation in critically ill patients in shock is the mainstay of therapy to maintain effective circulating blood volume. Timing of fluid resuscitation plays an important role in resuscitation and is based on the pathophysiology of shock [9, 10]. A long-standing controversy exists between proponents of colloids versus crystalloids for those patients. Supporters of crystalloids argue about risks of anaphylaxis, hemostasis impairment, and need for renal replacement therapy (RRT) with colloids as well as the potential to accumulate in tissues; whereas the colloid proponents argue with the risk of edema associated with crystalloids.

A recent Cochrane analysis concluded that there was no difference in mortality for hospitalized patients with trauma, burns, or following surgery when colloids were compared with crystalloids [11]. The use of HES may be associated with increased mortality; when they are compared to crystalloids, there was a higher incidence of adverse events and need for RRT [12, 13].

In the Crystalloid versus Hydroxyethyl Starch Trial (CHEST), involving 7000 adults in the ICU, the use of 6% HES (130/0.4), as compared with 0.9NS, was not associated with a significant difference in the rate of death at 90 days.

However, there was an increase in the rate of RRT and more adverse events in HES group [12]. The Colloids versus Crystalloids for the Resuscitation of the Critically Ill (CRISTAL) trial compared the effects of colloids versus crystalloids on mortality in patients presenting with hypovolemic shock [14]. There was no difference in mortality between the two groups at 28 days although 90-day mortality was lower in patients receiving colloids.

Low albumin levels are associated with all-cause mortality in both medical and surgical patients [15, 16]. Contrary to the belief that using albumin as a resuscitation fluid could improve mortality, a Cochrane review of 24 studies involving a total of 1419 patients, suggested that administration of albumin-containing fluids resulted in a 6% increase in the absolute risk of death when compared with use of crystalloid solutions [17]. This lead to the SAFE trial that showed similar outcomes between albumin and 0.9NS for resuscitation [18] No trial has consistently revealed superiority of albumin over crystalloids as resuscitative fluid.

In summary, there is no advantage of colloids versus crystalloids or vice versa. Considering the cost and adverse effect profile of colloids, crystalloids may be preferred over colloids. When colloids are used, care must be taken not to exceed recommended dose by regulatory agencies and avoid their use in patients with renal failure.

2.2. Question 2: are balanced fluids better than "0.9 normal saline?"

Normal saline is also referred as physiological or isotonic saline, neither of which is accurate. The sodium and chloride concentration of 154 mEq/L and the pH of 5.6 are certainly abnormal in "normal saline." The strong ion difference (SID) is the difference between the positively- and negatively-charged strong ions in plasma. Disturbances that increase the SID increase the blood pH while disorders that decrease the SID lower the plasma pH. This may also occur with volume resuscitation with 0.9NS (>30 cc/kg/h) due to excessive chloride administration impairing bicarbonate resorption in the kidneys resulting in hyperchloremic metabolic acidosis [19]. Other potential effects of 0.9NS include renal vasoconstriction with worsening renal function [20], increased postoperative complications, coagulation abnormalities [21], and an increased risk of death [22–24].

Lactated ringer, Plasma-Lyte, and Normosol are often called 'balanced fluids' as their electrolyte contents are closer to human plasma. These balanced crystalloids are also nearly isotonic but have a chloride concentration less than 110 mEq/L and a SID close to plasma.

Several trials comparing 0.9NS to balanced fluids have reported multiple outcomes. Outcomes have ranged from renal failure to mortality. Among critically ill adults with sepsis, resuscitation with balanced fluids was associated with a lower risk of in-hospital mortality [25]. In a meta-analysis of 11 RCTs (8 trials in operation room and 3 in ICU) involving 2703 patients, the in-hospital mortality, occurrence of acute kidney injury (AKI), and need for RRT was not different between balanced solutions and 0.9NS, irrespective of the location of the patients [26]. In a before and after trial comparing 0.9NS with LR solution, use of saline was a safe, viable alternative to LR in the trauma population [27]. In ICU patients requiring crystalloid fluid therapy, the use of a buffered crystalloid compared with saline did not reduce the risk of AKI or mortality [28]. Data regarding best fluid for the perioperative period is still inconclusive [29]. In patients undergoing renal transplants, balanced electrolyte solutions were associated with less hyperchloremic metabolic acidosis compared to 0.9NS, but there were no difference in graft outcomes [30]. Among critically ill adults, the use of balanced crystalloids for IVF administration resulted in a lower rate of the composite outcome of death from any cause, new RRT or persistent renal dysfunction when compared to 0.9NS [31] Among noncritically ill adults treated with IVFs in the emergency department, there was no difference in hospital-free days between treatment with balanced crystalloids compared with saline [32].

Some myths about Ringers lactate:

1. *Ringers lactate in renal failure*: In a study comparing acid-base status in kidney transplant patients, LR compared with 0.9NS may lead to a lower serum potassium level and a lower risk of acidosis [33]. In a randomized, double-blind comparison of LR's solution and 0.9%NS during renal transplantation, LR was associated with less hyperkalemia and acidosis compared with 0.9NS [34].
2. *Ringers lactate in hepatic failure*: LR is avoided in patients with hepatic failure with the fear of inducing or worsening lactic acidosis. However, lactate is given as sodium lactate, which is a base rather than an acid. There are no data describing LR causing worse outcomes compared to saline in patients with hepatic dysfunction.

In summary, 0.9%NS is not superior to balanced fluids in volume resuscitation in both critically ill and noncritically ill patients, perioperative patients and posttrauma. Studies suggest that use of balanced crystalloids for IVF administration results in a lower rate of the composite outcome of death from any cause, new RRT, or persistent renal dysfunction than the use of 0.9%NS in critically ill patients. Balanced fluids are not harmful compared to 0.9%NS and seem to be the fluid of choice. However, caution is advised when balanced solutions are used in patients with renal failure and hyperkalemia. Normal saline is an ideal choice in patients with metabolic alkalosis and chloride deficits who are vomiting or have nasogastric tube to suction.

2.3. Question 3: what are the common indications for hypertonic saline?

The classical indication for 3% saline is symptomatic severe hyponatremia. This is discussed in detail later in this chapter. Other indication for hypertonic saline is resuscitation in patients with traumatic brain injury (TBI). In patients with TBI, osmotic agents to reduce cerebral edema are recommended [35]. Common osmotic agents are mannitol and hypertonic saline. Hypertonic saline decreases intracranial pressure (ICP), improves microcirculation, and acts as anti-inflammatory [36]. A retrospective study comparing effectiveness of mannitol versus hypertonic saline revealed that hypertonic saline given in boluses may be more effective than mannitol in lowering ICP but no difference was found in short-term mortality [37]. A comparison of effects in coagulation function or increase in the risk of intracranial rebleeding in patients with moderate TBI when using 3% hypertonic saline versus 20% mannitol for the control of ICP showed no differences [38]. A comparison of pharmacologic therapeutic agents used for the reduction of intracranial pressure after traumatic brain injury concluded that hypertonic saline exhibits beneficial advantages compared with the other medications as a first-line treatment of intracranial hypertension in patients with severe TBI [39]. Complications of hypertonic saline use include hypernatremia, hyperchloremia, and renal failure. Mannitol and hypertonic saline in equiosmolar concentrations produced comparable effects on ICP reduction, brain relaxation, and systemic hemodynamic [40].

Hypertonic saline has been advocated in patients with volume loss after trauma, whereas TBI seems to be an indication to decrease cerebral edema, use of hypertonic saline in other situations is still unclear. In a meta-analysis, use of hypertonic saline showed no differences in clinical outcomes for hypotensive injured patients compared to isotonic fluid in the prehospital setting [41]. There is no evidence that hypertonic saline provides any additional benefit over isotonic crystalloid solutions for trauma resuscitation [42].

In summary, hypertonic saline can be used to decrease intra cranial pressure in patients with moderate to severe TBI. Care must be taken to avoid hypernatremia, hyperchloremia, and renal failure.

2.4. Question 4: how do we manage fluids in sepsis and septic shock?

In severe sepsis and septic shock, early volume resuscitation is indicated to save lives [43–45]; however, the best choice of fluids is unclear.

In a multicenter ICU trial of patients with severe sepsis randomly assigned to either 6% HES 130/0.42 or ringers acetate, patients receiving 6% HES 130/0.42 had a significant increase in the rate of death at 90 days and need for RRT. Several meta-analyses have shown that albumin does not provide a mortality benefit or decrease the need for RRT in critically ill patients, including those with hypoalbuminemia and sepsis [46–48]. A recent trial comparing albumin in addition to crystalloids versus crystalloids alone did not confer survival benefit in patients with severe sepsis or septic shock [49].

The early 2000s saw a resurgence in the use of hypertonic saline for sepsis resuscitation. Small volume resuscitation with hypertonic saline was postulated to achieve hemodynamic normalization by recruitment of fluid from the intracellular space, limiting interstitial edema [50]. Additional advantages included improved microcirculatory flow and favorable immunomodulatory effects. Two clinical trials have investigated the use of hypertonic saline in adult septic patients and there was no mortality difference [51, 52].

In the risk-adjusted inverse probability weighting analyses including 60,734 adults admitted to 360 ICUs across the United States between January 2006 and December 2010, the hospital mortality was 17.7% in the balanced fluid group, 19.2% in the 0.9%NS plus balanced fluids plus colloid group, 20.2% in the 0.9NS group ,and 24.2% in the saline plus colloid group. Balanced crystalloids were consistently associated with lower mortality. The authors concluded that when compared with exclusive use of 0.9%NS during resuscitation, coadministration of balanced crystalloids is associated with lower in-hospital mortality and no difference in LOS or costs per day. When colloids are coadministered, LOS and costs per day are increased without improved survival [53].

In summary, balanced fluids may be preferred over 0.9%NS in the resuscitation of patients with severe sepsis or septic shock without renal/liver or potassium issues. Hypertonic saline and other colloids including albumin are likely of no benefit over crystalloids. Use of starch is associated with adverse effects including increased need for RRT.

2.5. Question 5: fluid management in diabetic ketoacidosis

Patients with diabetic ketoacidosis (DKA) present with high anion gap metabolic acidosis, dehydration, and fluid deficits. Caution is advised in use of 0.9%NS due to two reasons. First, cerebral edema is a risk factor for death in patients with DKA. When a saline bolus is administered, it will distribute initially in the plasma that reaches the blood-brain barrier before equilibrating with the extracellular compartment. This has the potential to increase the interstitial volume of the brain ECF compartment and leads to cerebral edema. Second, chloride load in 0.9%NS can trigger nonanion gap metabolic acidosis.

A large bolus of 0.9%NS should be given only in emergent situations. It is advised to limit the amount of sodium ions infused in the first 120 min of therapy to about 3 mmol/kg body weight.

In a multicenter retrospective analysis of adults admitted for DKA to the ICU, which received almost exclusively Plasma-Lyte or 0.9%NS infusion up to 12 h, patients with PL had faster initial resolution of metabolic acidosis and less hyperchloremia, with a transiently improved blood pressure profile and urine output [54].

In summary: caution should be used using 0.9%NS in DKA and it is prudent to limit its use. If continued fluid resuscitation is needed, choice of fluids should be based on sNa levels. In patients with eunatremia or hypernatremia 0.45%NS is preferred and should be infused at 4–14 ml/kg/h, 0.9%NS is preferred in hyponatremia patients [55, 56].

2.6. Question 6: does my patient need maintenance fluids?

Maintenance fluid therapy is indicated in patients who are unable to eat for prolonged period of time in order to provide for fluids, electrolytes, and possibly some nutrition. The goal is to provide enough fluid and electrolytes to meet insensible losses and enable renal excretion of waste products. On an average, 2500 ml of water is ingested daily of which 60% is in form of fluids. Maintenance fluids should be a short-term measure since inappropriate therapy risks volume overload and electrolyte and acid-base disturbance. It is recommended to use 25–30 ml/kg/day water, 1 mmol/kg/day sodium, potassium, chloride, and 50–100 g/day glucose daily [57].

Higher insensible losses and hence higher maintenance of fluids needs to be considered in patients with ongoing losses, fever, burns, and third space losses especially in post-operative surgical patients. There is no evidence to use one kind of crystalloids over the other, hypotonic solutions should be avoided to avoid hyponatremia and avoidance of excessive sodium overload with 0.9%NS. Monitoring and avoidance of development of electrolyte imbalance is critical. Daily weights will prevent volume overload. Continuation of maintenance fluids should be critically reviewed in a daily bases.

2.7. Question 7: is there an ideal IV fluid?

An ideal resuscitative fluid should have an electrolyte composition close to plasma, should not accumulate in tissue, and must be completely metabolized. An ideal fluid does not exist and fluids should be treated as any other medication—indications, duration, effects, and adverse effects. Deciding which fluids are appropriate for each patient depends on the type of fluid lost and the body compartment(s) that require additional volume. It is advisable to consider patients comorbid conditions, acid-base and electrolyte status, and the indication for fluids before making a final selection. Timing of therapy is based on clinical context, delayed resuscitation is not only resuscitation denied but could have a detrimental effect.

Education of use of fluids to the health care providers, especially those who usually initiate care on hospital admission is paramount to improve outcomes and decrease morbidity and mortality.

Pearls:

1. Treat IVF like medications and consider risks, benefits, alternatives, and risks of alternatives.
2. In most instances, balanced solutions may be adequate.
3. Normal saline is probably the fluid of choice in patients with metabolic alkalosis due to vomiting or gastrointestinal losses with volume and chloride deficits.
4. In critically ill adults, the use of 0.9%NS for IVF administration results in a higher rate of the composite outcome of death from any cause, new RRT, or persistent renal dysfunction.
5. In patients with DKA, use of 0.9%NS should be restricted to 1–1.5 L unless a compelling indication.
6. Hypertonic saline or colloids are fluids of choice in TBI with cerebral edema.
7. Role of hypertonic saline in trauma other than TBI, severe sepsis, septic shock, and hemorrhagic shock is uncertain.
8. HES is a risk factor for renal injury and need for RRT.
9. If a synthetic colloid is chosen, do not exceed the manufacturer recommended maximal dose.
10. Use maintenance fluids only when indicated and review need daily.

3. Disorders of sodium imbalance

3.1. Hyponatremia

3.1.1. Question 8: what is the importance of hyponatremia?

Hyponatremia is a common laboratory abnormality; it is usually defined as a sNa of less than 136 mmol/L. The sNa cut offs to define hyponatremia varies from 125 to 135 mmol/L depending on different studies [58, 59].

Hyponatremia have been reported in 8% of the general population and in up to 60% of hospitalized patients [60]. Patients in ambulatory setting have a lower rate compared with hospital or skill nursing facility setting. Miller et al. reported an 11% incidence of hyponatremia in the ambulatory setting among elderly population with a median age of 78 years [61, 62].

The importance of hyponatremia is related not only to the absolute sNa value, but to the underlying conditions leading to it; it can be the tip of a serious condition. Severity of hyponatremia or its management can impact the patient's outcomes. Hyponatremia is not a disease, but a manifestation of an underlying disorder. The main focus of the management of hyponatremia is to elucidate the etiology and correction of laboratory abnormalities when levels are life threatening [59, 63].

Two major international guidelines attempted to address best practices in the management of this condition. The United States guidelines were published in 2013, however, they did not include grade of evidence due to scarce clinical evidence and resorted to expert panel recommendations [64]. In 2014, the European guidelines were published and included quality of evidence grades [65–67]. Rather than the absolute value of the sNa levels, the acuity of development of hyponatremia and its correction are of prime importance because the rate of change in sNa levels is associated with mortality, morbidity, and LOS [68, 69]. Mortality associated with hyponatremia has been reported as high as 30% [69].

A summary of relevant publications addressing prevalence of hyponatremia can be seen in **Table 3**. The serum cut off values for sodium in all those studies was between 130 and 138 and most of the studies were randomized control studies [58, 59].

3.2. Classification

Hyponatremia can be classified based in:

- Severity: this is based only in the absolute level of sNa. Mild 130–135 mmol/L, moderate 125–130 mmol/L, and severe when sNA is lower than 125 mmol/L.
- Time interval of development: acute-less than 48 h and chronic if more than 48 h. This information is occasionally difficult to obtain, but causes are usually different for acute and chronic hyponatremia.
- Measured osmolarity: it is fundamental to differentiate between the true hypotonic state from the isotonic and hypertonic state. Isotonic hyponatremia is usually due to pseudohyponatremia secondary to high plasma concentrations of triglycerides or proteins [70]. Expected changes in sNa in hypertriglyceridemia (TG) can be calculated as TG × 0.0002 = decrease in sNa in mEq/L; for plasma proteins (PP), PP in gm/dl – 8 × 0.25 = decrease in sNa in mEq/L.

  Commonest causes of hypertonic hyponatremia are hyperglycemia, administration of mannitol or other agents; the osmotic shift of water from ICF to ECF increases the total plasma volume diluting the sNa levels. Each increase in serum glucose levels by every 100 mg/dl after 150 mg/dl, decreases the sNa by approximately 1.6 mmol/L [71].
- Volume status: hypovolemia, euvolemia, and hypervolemia [72]. This is the most common classification used in the United States [64]. However, this classification is intrinsically flawed as there are no reliable, readily available and highly sensitive clinical tools to differentiate volume status, especially to differentiate hypovolemia from euvolemia [73–75]. Euvolemia itself is considered to be a misnomer as loss of sodium cannot happen without loss of water [2]. Clinical assessment is more reliable in cases of hypervolemia [2].

  Erroneous classification of patients into these categories can have detrimental outcomes [76].

Reference	Frequency (%)	Sample size	Outcome
Ambulatory setting			
Hawkins et al.	0.14	24,027	NA
Liamis et al.	7.7	5179	↑ Mortality
Gankam Kengne et al.	6	3551	↑ Mortality
Mohan et al.	2.5	14,697	NA
Hospital			
Hawkins et al.	42.6	43,249	NA
Hoorn et al.	30	5437	NA
Wald et al.	30	34,761	↑ Mortality
Wakar et al.	14.5	98,411	↑ Mortality
Congestive heart failure			
Gheorghiade	20	47,647	↑ Mortality
Liver cirrhosis			
Angeli et al.	49	997	↑ Mortality
Dawas	11	5152	↑ Mortality
HIV infection			
Tang	38	259	↑ Mortality
Cusano et al.	31	96	↑ Mortality
Non-dialysis kidney failure			
Covesdy et al.	13	655,493	↑ Mortality
Pneumonia			
Zilberberg et al.	8	7965	↑ Mortality
Modified from [58, 59].			

Table 3. Prevalence and outcome of hyponatremia.

3.3. Clinical features

Symptoms of hyponatremia are initially subtle, nonspecifics, and difficult to recognize. They mostly manifest as neurological changes, which ranges from altered personality, lethargy and confusion to seizures, coma and death in severe cases [2, 77]. Symptomatic differences between acute severe and chronic hyponatremia have been reported. Symptoms of acute severe hyponatremia include nausea, vomiting, headache, seizure, coma, respiratory failure, and death, which are manifestations of brain edema. In chronic hyponatremia, main symptoms are fatigue, gait and attention deficit, osteoporosis, and fractures. Nausea and vomiting are seen in both, acute severe and chronic hyponatremia [78, 79]. Older patients with comorbid conditions tend to develop symptoms of hyponatremia at an earlier onset than young healthier patients. Premenopausal women are prone for cerebral edema from acute hyponatremia, it is hypothesized that this could be secondary to the action of estrogen and progesterone inhibiting Na+K+-ATPase and decreasing solute expel from brain cells; if not recognized early, it will lead to neurological complications. The nonneurological manifestations are often due to the dysregulation in the volume status [5, 80].

3.3.1. *Question 9: what are the causes of hyponatremia?*

The best approach to evaluate causes of hyponatremia is to first decide if we are dealing with acute versus chronic hyponatremia.

Acute hyponatremia: the underlying etiological mechanism primarily causes large input of water. Normal individuals with intact thirst center and mental function develop aversion to large volume water intake. **Table 4** shows most common causes of acute hyponatremia.

Chronic hyponatremia: slow onset of hyponatremia, usually more than 48 h. The underlying etiology is lower rate of water excretion and involves release of vasopressin. In some case, decreased volume of filtered solute and residual water permeability play a role [5]. **Table 5** shows most common causes of chronic hyponatremia and **Table 6** shows the most common laboratory findings in the most common causes of hypotonic hyponatremia.

3.3.2. *Question 10: how we evaluate a patient with hyponatremia?*

Evaluation of hyponatremia still remains to some extent controversial and occasionally cumbersome.

In an attempt to avoid the pitfalls of volume evaluation recommended in the 2012 guidelines, the European guidelines were released in 2014. They prioritized the use of urine sodium (uNa) levels and urine osmolality (uOsm) over assessment of volume status [67]. Conditions leading to a false low or high uNa levels like low sodium diet or recent diuretic use and chronic kidney disease respectively were addressed [66, 81, 82].

Role of vasopressin and copeptin levels: measurement of vasopressin levels seems logical for the investigation of hyponatremia, but its unstable nature when not bound to plasma, low accuracy, and not readily available makes it use unsuitable. Moreover, uOsm is a readily available, accurate, and inexpensive surrogate [83]. Vasopressin is degraded into neurophysin and copeptin by enzymatic cleavage. Copeptin has been considered also a reasonable surrogate for

Ingestion of large volume of water	Infusion of large volume of 5% dextrose	Infusion of large volume of hypotonic lavage fluid	Generation and retention of electrolyte-free water ("desalination")
• Mood-altering drugs which blocks aversion to large water intake • Increased water intake to avoid dehydration • Beer potomania • Psychotic state	• Postoperative period (especially patients with a low muscle mass)	• Input of water and organic solutes, with little or no Na+ ions (e.g. post transurethral resection of prostate)	• Excretion of large volume of hypertonic urine caused by a large infusion of isotonic saline in a setting where vasopressin is present

Table 4. Causes of acute hyponatremia.

http://dx.doi.org/10.5772/intechopen.79121

Lower rate of water excretion due to low volume of distal delivery of filtrate	Lower rate of water excretion due to vasopressin actions
• Very low glomerular filtration rate states • States with enhanced reabsorption of filtrate in the proximal collecting tubules caused by low effective arterial blood volume • Loss of Na+ and Cl− • Sweat: cystic fibrosis, marathon runner • Gastrointestinal tract: diarrhea • Renal: diuretics, aldosterone deficiency, renal or cerebral salt wasting • States with expanded extracellular fluid volume but low effective arterial blood volume (e.g., congestive heart failure, liver cirrhosis)	• Non-osmotic stimuli: pain, anxiety, nausea • Baroreceptor-mediated release of vasopressin due to very low EABV • Central stimulation of vasopressin: drugs like 3,4-methylenedioxymethamphetamine (MDMA), nicotine, morphine, carbamazepine, tricyclic antidepressants, serotonin reuptake inhibitors, antineoplastic agents • Pulmonary disorders: bacterial or viral pneumonia, tuberculosis • Central nervous system disorders: encephalitis, meningitis, brain tumors, subdural hematoma, subarachnoid hemorrhage, stroke • Release of vasopressin from malignant cells: small-cell carcinoma of the lung, oropharyngeal carcinomas, olfactory neuroblastomas • Administration of desmopressin • Glucocorticoid deficiency • Severe hypothyroidism • Activating mutation of the vasopressin 2 receptor: nephrogenic syndrome of inappropriate antidiuresis

Modified from [5].

Table 5. Causes of chronic hyponatremia.

Volume status	Clinical conditions	Urine Osm	Urine Na	Serum uric acid	FE_{NA}
Hypovolemic (appropriate ADH response)	Extrarenal losses	Elevated	<10–20	Elevated >4	<1
	Renal losses deficiency of mineralocorticoids	Elevated	>20	Elevated	>1
Hypervolemic (appropriate ADH response)	Heart failure, liver cirrhosis, nephrotic syndrome	Elevated	<20	Low/normal	<1
	Renal failure	Decreased	>20	Variable	>1
Euvolemia	Reset osmostat	Variable			
	SIADH	Elevated >100–300	>30–40	Decreased <4	>1
	Primary polydipsia	Decreased	Decreased	Low/normal	>1
	Hypothyroidism, deficiency of mineralocorticoids	Elevated	>20	Low/normal	>1

Table 6. Laboratory findings in most common causes of hypotonic hyponatremia.

vasopressin. Copeptin levels were reported to be increased in hypo and hypervolemic hyponatremia but not in syndrome of inappropriate secretion of antidiuretic hormone (SIADH). A ratio of serum copeptin to uNa with a cut off value of 30 pmol/mmol had an AUC of 0.88 in identifying hypovolemia from euvolemia [84].

Other biomarkers like apelin and midregional proatrial natriuretic peptide (MR-ProANP) have been evaluated in hyponatremia. Apelin counteract vasopressin in homeostasis. MR-ProANP increases to a larger extent in hypo or hypervolemic hyponatremia rather than in SIADH. The true diagnostic potential of these biomarkers are yet to be validated [85–88].

Based on existing guidelines and trying to overcome limitations of clinical evaluation of volume status, we suggest the following steps when evaluating a patient with hyponatremia:

1. Measurement of serum osmolarity to differentiate between hypotonic hyponatremia from iso- and hypertonic.
2. Hypotonic hyponatremia: clinical evaluation of volume status. In general, identification of hypervolemia is more accurate than differentiating between euvolemic and hypovolemic state.
3. Measurement of urine osmolarity (uOsm) and urinary sodium (uNa). This is conjunction with sOsm and examination should narrow down the diagnosis. For example, a threshold of uOsm of >100 mOsm/kg predicts the action of ADH on the collecting tubules, which in case of hyponatremia is not the appropriate response. This together with elevated uNa >20–30 mmol/L strongly suggests the presence of SIADH [2].
4. Needs to consider the presence of more than one disorder leading to hyponatremia [89].
5. Management should ideally address correction of sNa levels as well as the underlying condition leading to it.
6. Delayed or unavailability of sOsm is one of the major limiting factors during evaluation of hyponatremia as addressed by the United States guidelines, potentially leading to misclassification of patients based on clinical assessment of volume status.
7. Some experts suggest that a limited work up including sOsm, uNa, uOsm, and infusion of isotonic saline 1–2 l over 24 h may be sufficient for an accurate diagnosis in most cases of hypotonic hyponatremia [2]. Increase in sNa after trial of volume expansion suggests hypovolemic hyponatremia. However, this can be also seen in SIADH [75, 90–92].

Volume expansion should be cautiously done in certain conditions like immediate post-operative period, where isotonic saline can worsen the hyponatremia by a process called desalination, as presence of vasopressin makes the urine hypertonic by water resorption [93]. In addition, patients with hypervolemic states like heart failure or liver cirrhosis could deteriorate with the additional fluid administration.

Figure 1 shows a flow diagram for initial evaluation of hyponatremia.

3.3.3. Question 11: how do we manage hyponatremia?

Goal should ideally focus in the prevention of hyponatremia knowing its association with significant morbidity and mortality. There is no data available regarding the effects of treating asymptomatic mild to moderate hyponatremia [2, 94, 95].

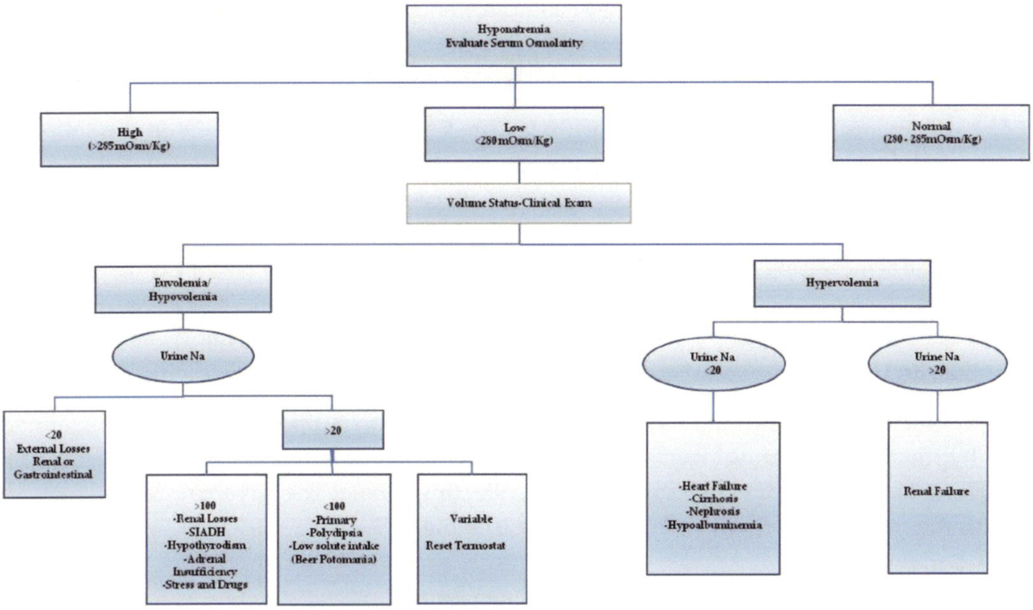

Figure 1. Algorithm for initial evaluation of hyponatremia. Based in the USA and European guidelines [64–67].

Patients presenting with severe, acute, or chronic hyponatremia should be treated in a monitor setting as those patients are at risk for adverse outcomes [2]. Acute respiratory failure from damage of the respiratory center or noncardiogenic pulmonary edema has been reported [96, 97]. Identification of patients at higher risk for osmotic demyelination remains a challenge during treatment; risks factors for development of osmotic demyelination include presence hypokalemia, alcoholism, malnutrition, and liver disease [64, 98]. **Table 7** shows basic management of patients presenting with hyponatremia and comparison of the two major existing guidelines.

Areas of concern with guidelines: caution must be excised when following guidelines. Areas of concern in the management of hyponatremia are:

- There is no clear evidence regarding the 48 h cut off to differentiate between acute and chronic hyponatremia, neither to clearly differentiate risk for osmotic demyelination in those patients.
- Clinically difficult to be certain regarding acuity of hyponatremia; in asymptomatic patients with hyponatremia, it could be assumed to be chronic.
- Limited evidence regarding the best and safer correction rate. A lower correction rate of 6 mEq/L/24 h could be safer.
- When to treat a patient with mild to moderate hyponatremia and none/minimal neurological symptoms remain a gray zone and depends on the clinical situation. Fluid restriction is the most common, cost effective, and safer modality of treatment [2, 72]. Fluid restriction of 500–1000 ml/day has been suggested and should be based in volume assessment. Urine Na to serum

electrolyte ratio (uNa + urine K/sNa) >1 indicates antidiuretic phase and a ratio <1 suggests aquaretic phase. Fluid restrictions to less than 500 ml/day in antidiuretic phase and 1000 ml/day in aquaretic phase have been recommended; however, adherence is a problem [72].

- Use of Vaptans. Vaptans are vasopressin type 2 receptor antagonist, present in the collecting duct and they induce excretion of hypotonic urine. Its use has been recommended in a subgroup of patients with hyponatremia secondary to excess vasopressin [99, 100]. There are many vaptans available including tolvaptan, satavaptan, lixivaptan, and conivaptan, which are been successful at increasing sNa and relieving symptoms in conditions like SIADH, congestive heart failure, and liver cirrhosis [101–103]. Sodium overcorrection is a concern and it was reported in 25% of 61 patients included in a study [103]. Side effects including liver injury, risk of overcorrection, and lack of long-term sodium improvement are some of limitations [101, 102, 104].
- Demeclocycline and lithium have low quality evidence to support front line management of hyponatremia. Demeclocycline is thought to inhibit adenylate cyclase activity upon binding of vasopressin to its receptor in the collecting tubule. The adverse effects associated with the drugs make them less desirable for treatment [2, 105].

3.3.4. Question 12: what are the complications and outcomes of hyponatremia?

Complications of hyponatremia can be divided in those caused by hyponatremia per se and those caused by the treatment of hyponatremia. In general, worse outcomes are associated with sNa levels of less than 115 mEq/L and with faster rate of fall in sNa [2].

3.4. Complications and outcomes of untreated hyponatremia

Complications of hyponatremia range from chronic debilitating symptoms like gait deficit and neuromuscular symptoms to a more severe and life-threatening presentation of brain edema. Chronic and mild-moderate hyponatremia have been associated with attention or gait deficits, increased risk of falls, and bone fractures. Bone is a reservoir for Na. Observational retrospective cross sectional and epidemiological surveys have established an association between chronic hyponatremia and osteoporosis and major osteoporotic fracture [106–111].

Unfortunately, there is a lack of evidence to suggest that osteoporosis is reversed with correction of hyponatremia [2].

The brain which is contained in the hard skull is not able to accommodate any swelling or increase in brain volume. This is evident especially in patients who develop acute hyponatremia. Cerebral edema occurs when cells within the brain swell, when there is an increase in extracellular fluid volume in the brain or both. Brain cells swell when there is a large osmotic force favoring an intracellular shift of water, owing to a higher effective osmolality in brain cells than the effective osmolality in plasma in capillaries near the blood–brain barrier [112–115]. The elevated intracranial pressure with the resultant acute cerebral edema can potentially lead to serious symptoms that ranges from seizures, coma to brain herniation causing irreversible midbrain damage and death [116, 117]. Incidence of fatal brain damage secondary to severe hyponatremia is unknown, majority of the cases have been reported during the perioperative period secondary to infusion of hypotonic fluids or self-water intoxication like marathon runners and psychiatric patients [118].

Conditions	General agreement in guidelines	Disagreement between guidelines
Acute or symptomatic hyponatremia—less 48 h	*Severe symptoms:* bolus 3% NaCl: 100–150 ml over 10–20 min × 2–3 as needed	Minimal—just in amount of fluids 50 ml difference
	Moderate symptoms: continuous infusion 3% NaCl 0.5–2 ml/kg/h or bolus 3% NaCl: 100–150 ml over 20 min × 1	
Chronic hyponatremia—more 48 h		
SIADH	First line: fluid restriction	None
	Second line: demeclocycline, urea, or vaptan	European guidelines do not recommend vaptans when sNa > 130 and recommend against when sNa > 125.
		Recommends against demeclocycline
		Suggest oral NaCl or loop diuretics
Hypovolemic hyponatremia	Isotonic saline or balanced crystalloid solution	Minimal/none
Hypervolemic hyponatremia	Fluid restriction—500—1 L/day Vaptans	European guidelines recommend against vaptan
Correction rates	Minimum-only USA guidelines: 4–8 mmol/L/day, 4–6 mmol/L/day in high risk of neurological complications	European guidelines have no minimum
	Limits: 10–12 mmol/L/day, 8 mmol/L/day in high risk patients	None
Management of overcorrection	Baseline sNa ≥ 120 mmol/L: probably unnecessary	European guidelines suggest to start once limit is exceeded
	Baseline sNa < 120 mmol/L: relower with electrolyte-free water or desmopressin after correction exceeds 6–8 mmol/L/day	Expert consultations recommended by European guidelines

Modified from [72].

Table 7. Management of hypotonic hyponatremia and comparison between existing guidelines.

Most cases of hyponatremia in the ambulatory setting are mild. An sNa of less than 125 mmol/L was seen in 0.14% in Hawkin et al. study [60]. The Dallas heart study, a large prospective multiethnic cohort study of 3551 ambulatory individuals with median age of 43 year/age and from diverse ethnicity, found that mild hyponatremia (median 133 mmol/L) was significantly associated with increased risk of death [119]. A large cross sectional observational study by the National Health and Nutrition Examination Survey in the United States with 15,000 individuals demonstrated that hyponatremia was an independent risk for increased mortality across age, gender, and comorbid conditions. Overall prevalence was around 2%. They also showed that prevalence of hyponatremia increased with age and was more frequent among women than men [120].

Others studies looking at the association of hyponatremia with specific comorbid conditions like heart failure, HIV, pneumonia, renal failure among others, concluded that hyponatremia is an independent risk factor for mortality regardless the levels of sNa [58, 121–129]. Among patients presenting with acute pulmonary emboli, hyponatremia is common and several studies has shown to be an independent risk factor for increased short-term mortality. This result could be encountered as a variable in determining of pulmonary emboli severity and mortality [130, 131].

Among the hospitalized population, many studies have estimated the prevalence of hyponatremia from 8 to 40% [60, 69, 89, 132]. In Wald et al. study evaluating more than 50,000 patients, he established that irrespective of onset of hyponatremia-community, hospital aggravated or hospital acquired, all were associated with increased mortality, length of stay, and discharge to a facility; and this was independent of the underlying comorbid conditions. Mortality was increased among older patients. The operational definition for normal sNa in this study was 138–142 mEq/L. In patients with hospital acquired hyponatremia, the risk of mortality was 15 times higher among patients with first serum sodium level of 127 mEq/L or less [69]. A larger prospective study by Waiker and colleagues with approximately 100,000 individuals followed up to 5 years showed that irrespective of the severity of hyponatremia, presence of hyponatremia independently increased risk of dead with an odd ratio of 1.47, 1.32, and 1.33 at the time of admission, 1 and 5 year follow-up, respectively. It was more pronounced among patients admitted with cardiovascular disease, metastatic cancer, and those admitted for procedures related to the musculoskeletal system. They also showed that resolution of hyponatremia attenuated the increased risk of mortality [132].

3.5. Complications and outcomes of treatment of hyponatremia

There are no many studies evaluating outcomes of treatment of hyponatremia. Two studies evaluated the impact of treatment on mortality among patients with congestive heart failure and concluded that treatment confers no mortality benefit, however, there was symptomatic improvement and decreased length of stay [94, 95]. Other studies suggested that correction of mild hyponatremia could reverse attention and gait deficits [133, 134].

When hyponatremia develops over a slower rate, 24–48 h, the brain cells are able to adapt to expel enough of anions and organic solutes along with water to maintain its size. Rapid correction of hyponatremia can lead to inability to regain the organic solutes causing osmotic demyelination, a process still poorly understood [5].

Osmotic demyelination syndrome (ODS) and central pontine myelinolysis (CPM) are terms usually used interchangeably, but they represent separate, not well understood and highly feared complications of the treatment of hyponatremia. The effect of rapid correction of hyponatremia is termed as ODS and it is specific to the central nervous system and not always localized to the pontine region. Extrapontine myelinolysis is as frequent as CPM [135, 136]. Risk factors making patients more susceptible to the development of ODS include severity and chronicity of hyponatremia, the increment of sNa, the treatment used for sodium correction, concomitant hypokalemia, presence of liver disease and the nutritional status [98]. A small study of 33 patients showed that an increase in sNa to normal or hypernatremic levels in the first 48 h, a change in the sNa concentration of >25 mmol/L in the first 48 h, a hypoxic-anoxic episode, and an elevation of sNa to hypernatremic levels in patients with hepatic encephalopathy were associated with CMP. However, rate of correction was not associated with demyelination [118].

The clinical manifestations of ODS are variable depending on the location of demyelination. They range from pontine and bulbar symptoms such as dysarthria, dysphagia, and dystonia to more severe forms like locked-in state and coma [137]. In the past, prognosis of ODS and CMP was considered to be very poor; however, several studies have reported near complete neurological recovery. In addition, ODS/CMP are associated with other complications like aspiration pneumonia, urinary tract infection, deep venous thrombosis, and pulmonary embolism [137–139].

3.6. How can ODS be avoided?

In the absence of an absolute threshold for the rate of correction, it is well accepted that the safest rate of correction of hyponatremia is 6–8 mEq/L/day. Brain demyelination has been reported over a range of rate of sNa correction of 8–12–18 mEq/L/day [2, 72]. Some investigators in small, nonrandomized studies suggest concomitant use of desmopressin and hypertonic saline for better control of the rate of sNa correction in hyponatremia [140, 141]. Experiments on rats have shown little success with the combination regimen of D5W and desmopressin for the treatment of overcorrection of hyponatremia [142, 143]. The role of urea for ODS have not been well studied.

3.7. Hypernatremia

A difference of the complexity of hyponatremia, the finding of hypernatremia invariably denotes hypertonic hyperosmolality and always causes cellular dehydration. It is usually defined as a sNa of more than 145 mmol/L. It can be a frequent finding in hospitalized patients or high risk patients with poor access to water like the elderly, infants, patients on mechanical ventilation, and patients with altered mental status. In the elderly, a physiologic decrease in the thirst mechanism have been reported; however, there can be a pathological decrease in free water intake as well [60].

In general, clinical manifestations of hypernatremia correlate with the severity of sodium abnormalities and are related to central nervous system dysfunction and ranges from weakness, confusion to seizure and coma. In addition, sign of hypovolemia and hemodynamic abnormalities can be found on examination.

The complications of hypernatremia vary from mild to life threatening [144]. Brain shrinkage induced by hypernatremia can cause vascular rupture, with cerebral bleeding, subarachnoid hemorrhage, and permanent neurologic damage or death.

Causes of hypernatremia can be loose classified in two: either net water losses due to gastrointestinal or renal etiologies or hypertonic solution administration [144, 145].

3.7.1. Management of hypernatremia

The focus of management is addressing the underlying cause leading to hypernatremia and the correction of serum sodium. Initial evaluation includes evaluation of vital signs. In hemodynamically unstable patients, administration of isotonic 0.9% normal saline or balance fluids is advised, irrespective of sNa. Goal in those patients is fluid resuscitation hemodynamic stabilization. Patient who are hemodynamically stable can be managed with oral or IVF replacement. The preferred route for fluid administration is the oral route or a feeding tube; otherwise IVF are required. Only hypotonic fluids are recommended, including pure water, 5% dextrose, and 0.2 or 0.45% sodium chloride. The more hypotonic the infusate, the lower the infusion rate required. An easy and efficient way to calculate this is by using Adrogue-Madias formula, which allows to calculate rate of infusate [144].

Correction rates: similar to management of hyponatremia, and to avoid sudden changes in tonicity, the target recommended fall in the sNa concentration is 8–10 mmol/L/day for patients with hypernatremia with a goal to reduce the sNa to 145 mmol/L [145, 146].

Pearls:

1. Serum sodium abnormalities are common and carry significant morbidity and mortality.
2. Evaluation of sodium abnormalities should focus in the underlying condition as well as management.
3. Following recommended algorithms for evaluation of hyponatremia is advised.
4. Evaluation of volume status in patients with sodium disorders can be a challenge.
5. Needs to keep in consideration the presence of more than one disorder.
6. Resuscitation of an unstable patient takes precedence over correction of sodium levels.
7. There is no rush to correct sNa levels, risk of overcorrection, or rapid increase in sNa can lead to serious complications.

4. Conclusion

We reviewed issues related to fluids and sodium disturbance and the clinical implications of these issues. The dysregulation of fluid and sodium homeostasis leads to many direct and indirect effects and carries significant morbidity and mortality in a wide variety of patients and clinical settings. Those range from mild cases of dehydration to more severe cases of patients in shock or with severe hypo- or hypernatremia.

Since the high prevalence of these disorders, clinicians in virtually every medical specialty will interact with patients requiring fluid administration and need for electrolyte evaluation and correction. Appropriate and timely administration of fluids and electrolyte correction with focus in avoidance of complications and improvement of outcomes is fundamental.

Conflict of interest

The authors have no conflict of interest.

http://dx.doi.org/10.5772/intechopen.79121

Abbreviations

ECF	extracellular fluid
ICF	intracellular fluid
IVF	intravenous fluids
RRT	renal replacement therapy
HES	hydroxyethyl starches
SID	strong ion difference
TBI	traumatic brain injury

Author details

Gilda Diaz-Fuentes[1,2]*, Bharat Bajantri[1,2] and Sindhaghatta Venkatram[1,2]

*Address all correspondence to: gfuentes@bronxleb.org

1 Division of Pulmonary Critical Care, Department of Medicine, BronxCare Health System, Bronx, New York, USA

2 Icahn School of Medicine at Mount Sinai, USA

References

[1] Watson PE, Watson ID, Batt RD. Total body water volumes for adult males and females estimated from simple anthropometric measurements. The American Journal of Clinical Nutrition. 1980;**33**(1):27-39

[2] Gankam Kengne F. Physiopathology, clinical diagnosis, and treatment of hyponatremia. Acta Clinica Belgica. 2016;**71**(6):359-372

[3] Farber SJ. Mucopolysaccharides and sodium metabolism. Circulation. 1960;**21**:941-947

[4] Forbes GB, Tobin RB, Harrison A, McCoord A. Effect of acute hypernatremia, hyponatremia, and acidosis on bone sodium. The American Journal of Physiology. 1965; **209**(4):825-829

[5] Kamel KS, Halperin ML. Chapter 10—Hyponatremia. In: Fluid, Electrolyte and Acid-Base Physiology. 5th ed. Philadelphia: Elsevier; 2017. pp. 265-308

[6] Sharif-Naeini R, Ciura S, Zhang Z, Bourque CW. Contribution of TRPV channels to osmosensory transduction, thirst, and vasopressin release. Kidney International. 2008; **73**(7):811-815

[7] Bichet DG, Arthus MF, Lonergan M, Hendy GN, Paradis AJ, Fujiwara TM, et al. X-linked nephrogenic diabetes insipidus mutations in North America and the Hopewell hypothesis. The Journal of Clinical Investigation. 1993;**92**(3):1262-1268

[8] Decaux G, Vandergheynst F, Bouko Y, Parma J, Vassart G, Vilain C. Nephrogenic syndrome of inappropriate antidiuresis in adults: High phenotypic variability in men and women from a large pedigree. Journal of the American Society of Nephrology. 2007;**18**(2):606-612

[9] Bickell WH, Wall MJ Jr, Pepe PE, Martin RR, Ginger VF, Allen MK, et al. Immediate versus delayed fluid resuscitation for hypotensive patients with penetrating torso injuries. The New England Journal of Medicine. 1994;**331**(17):1105-1109

[10] Rivers E, Nguyen B, Havstad S, Ressler J, Muzzin A, Knoblich B, et al. Early goal-directed therapy in the treatment of severe sepsis and septic shock. The New England Journal of Medicine. 2001;**345**(19):1368-1377

[11] Perel P, Roberts I, Ker K. Colloids versus crystalloids for fluid resuscitation in critically ill patients. Cochrane Database of Systematic Reviews. 2013;(2). DOI: 10.1002/14651858.CD000567.pub6

[12] Myburgh JA, Finfer S, Bellomo R, Billot L, Cass A, Gattas D, et al. Hydroxyethyl starch or saline for fluid resuscitation in intensive care. The New England Journal of Medicine. 2012;**367**(20):1901-1911

[13] Perner A, Haase N, Guttormsen AB, Tenhunen J, Klemenzson G, Aneman A, et al. Hydroxyethyl starch 130/0.42 versus Ringer's acetate in severe sepsis. The New England Journal of Medicine. 2012;**367**(2):124-134

[14] Annane D, Siami S, Jaber S, Martin C, Elatrous S, Declere AD, et al. Effects of fluid resuscitation with colloids vs crystalloids on mortality in critically ill patients presenting with hypovolemic shock: The CRISTAL randomized trial. Journal of the American Medical Association. 2013;**310**(17):1809-1817

[15] Gibbs J, Cull W, Henderson W, Daley J, Hur K, Khuri SF. Preoperative serum albumin level as a predictor of operative mortality and morbidity: Results from the National VA Surgical Risk Study. Archives of Surgery. 1999;**134**(1):36-42

[16] Jellinge ME, Henriksen DP, Hallas P, Brabrand M. Hypoalbuminemia is a strong predictor of 30day all-cause mortality in acutely admitted medical patients: A prospective, observational, cohort study. PLoS One. 2014;**9**(8):e105983

[17] Cochrane Injuries Group Albumin R. Human albumin administration in critically ill patients: Systematic review of randomised controlled trials. BMJ. 1998;**317**(7153):235-240

[18] Finfer S, Bellomo R, Boyce N, French J, Myburgh J, Norton R, et al. A comparison of albumin and saline for fluid resuscitation in the intensive care unit. The New England Journal of Medicine. 2004;**350**(22):2247-2256

[19] Park M, Calabrich A, Maciel AT, Zampieri FG, Taniguchi LU, Souza CE, et al. Physicochemical characterization of metabolic acidosis induced by normal saline resuscitation of patients with severe sepsis and septic shock. Revista Brasileira de Terapia Intensiva. 2011;**23**(2):176-182

[20] Yunos NM, Bellomo R, Hegarty C, Story D, Ho L, Bailey M. Association between a chloride-liberal vs chloride-restrictive intravenous fluid administration strategy and kidney injury in critically ill adults. Journal of the American Medical Association. 2012; **308**(15):1566-1572

[21] Waters JH, Gottlieb A, Schoenwald P, Popovich MJ, Sprung J, Nelson DR. Normal saline versus lactated Ringer's solution for intraoperative fluid management in patients undergoing abdominal aortic aneurysm repair: An outcome study. Anesthesia and Analgesia. 2001;**93**(4):817-822

[22] Shaw AD, Bagshaw SM, Goldstein SL, Scherer LA, Duan M, Schermer CR, et al. Major complications, mortality, and resource utilization after open abdominal surgery: 0.9% saline compared to Plasma-Lyte. Annals of Surgery. 2012;**255**(5):821-829

[23] Shaw AD, Raghunathan K, Peyerl FW, Munson SH, Paluszkiewicz SM, Schermer CR. Association between intravenous chloride load during resuscitation and in-hospital mortality among patients with SIRS. Intensive Care Medicine. 2014;**40**(12):1897-1905

[24] Magder S. Balanced versus unbalanced salt solutions: What difference does it make? Best Practice & Research. Clinical Anaesthesiology. 2014;**28**(3):235-247

[25] Raghunathan K, Shaw A, Nathanson B, Sturmer T, Brookhart A, Stefan MS, et al. Association between the choice of IV crystalloid and in-hospital mortality among critically ill adults with sepsis. Critical Care Medicine. 2014;**42**(7):1585-1591

[26] Serpa Neto A, Martin Loeches I, Klanderman RB, Freitas Silva R, Gama de Abreu M, Pelosi P, et al. Balanced versus isotonic saline resuscitation—A systematic review and meta-analysis of randomized controlled trials in operation rooms and intensive care units. Annals of Translational Medicine. 2017;**5**(16):323

[27] Davis JS, Alsafran S, Richie CD, Moore JW, Namias N, Schulman CI. Time to resuscitate a sacred cow…with normal saline. The American Surgeon. 2014;**80**(3):301-306

[28] Young P, Bailey M, Beasley R, Henderson S, Mackle D, McArthur C, et al. Effect of a buffered crystalloid solution vs saline on acute kidney injury among patients in the intensive care unit: The SPLIT randomized clinical trial. Journal of the American Medical Association. 2015;**314**(16):1701-1710

[29] Bampoe S, Odor PM, Dushianthan A, Bennett-Guerrero E, Cro S, Gan TJ, et al. Perioperative administration of buffered versus non-buffered crystalloid intravenous fluid to improve outcomes following adult surgical procedures. Cochrane Database of Systematic Reviews. 2017;**9**:CD004089

[30] Wan S, Roberts MA, Mount P. Normal saline versus lower-chloride solutions for kidney transplantation. Cochrane Database of Systematic Reviews. 2016;**8**:CD010741

[31] Semler MW, Self WH, Wanderer JP, Ehrenfeld JM, Wang L, Byrne DW, et al. Balanced crystalloids versus saline in critically ill adults. The New England Journal of Medicine. 2018;**378**(9):829-839

[32] Self WH, Semler MW, Wanderer JP, Wang L, Byrne DW, Collins SP, et al. Balanced crystalloids versus saline in noncritically ill adults. The New England Journal of Medicine. 2018;**378**(9):819-828

[33] Khajavi MR, Etezadi F, Moharari RS, Imani F, Meysamie AP, Khashayar P, et al. Effects of normal saline vs. lactated ringer's during renal transplantation. Renal Failure. 2008; **30**(5):535-539

[34] O'Malley CM, Frumento RJ, Hardy MA, Benvenisty AI, Brentjens TE, Mercer JS, et al. A randomized, double-blind comparison of lactated Ringer's solution and 0.9% NaCl during renal transplantation. Anesthesia and Analgesia. 2005;**100**(5):1518-1524 table of contents

[35] Carney N, Totten AM, O'Reilly C, Ullman JS, Hawryluk GW, Bell MJ, et al. Guidelines for the management of severe traumatic brain injury, fourth edition. Neurosurgery. 2017;**80**(1):6-15

[36] de Oliveira MF, Pinto FC. Hypertonic saline: A brief overview of hemodynamic response and antiinflammatory properties in head injury. Neural Regeneration Research. 2015; **10**(12):1938-1939

[37] Mangat HS, Chiu YL, Gerber LM, Alimi M, Ghajar J, Hartl R. Hypertonic saline reduces cumulative and daily intracranial pressure burdens after severe traumatic brain injury. Journal of Neurosurgery. 2015;**122**(1):202-210

[38] Wang H, Cao H, Zhang X, Ge L, Bie L. The effect of hypertonic saline and mannitol on coagulation in moderate traumatic brain injury patients. The American Journal of Emergency Medicine. 2017;**35**(10):1404-1407

[39] Alnemari AM, Krafcik BM, Mansour TR, Gaudin D. A comparison of pharmacologic therapeutic agents used for the reduction of intracranial pressure after traumatic brain injury. World Neurosurgery. 2017;**106**:509-528

[40] Sokhal N, Rath GP, Chaturvedi A, Singh M, Dash HH. Comparison of 20% mannitol and 3% hypertonic saline on intracranial pressure and systemic hemodynamics. Journal of Clinical Neuroscience. 2017;**42**:148-154

[41] Blanchard IE, Ahmad A, Tang KL, Ronksley PE, Lorenzetti D, Lazarenko G, et al. The effectiveness of prehospital hypertonic saline for hypotensive trauma patients: A systematic review and meta-analysis. BMC Emergency Medicine. 2017;**17**(1):35

[42] Patanwala AE, Amini A, Erstad BL. Use of hypertonic saline injection in trauma. American Journal of Health-System Pharmacy. 2010;**67**(22):1920-1928

[43] Mouncey PR, Osborn TM, Power GS, Harrison DA, Sadique MZ, Grieve RD, et al. Trial of early, goal-directed resuscitation for septic shock. The New England Journal of Medicine. 2015;**372**(14):1301-1311

[44] Pro CI, Yealy DM, Kellum JA, Huang DT, Barnato AE, Weissfeld LA, et al. A randomized trial of protocol-based care for early septic shock. The New England Journal of Medicine. 2014;**370**(18):1683-1693

[45] Investigators A, Group ACT, Peake SL, Delaney A, Bailey M, Bellomo R, et al. Goal-directed resuscitation for patients with early septic shock. The New England Journal of Medicine. 2014;**371**(16):1496-1506

[46] Patel A, Laffan MA, Waheed U, Brett SJ. Randomised trials of human albumin for adults with sepsis: Systematic review and meta-analysis with trial sequential analysis of all-cause mortality. BMJ. 2014;**349**:g4561

[47] Xu JY, Chen QH, Xie JF, Pan C, Liu SQ, Huang LW, et al. Comparison of the effects of albumin and crystalloid on mortality in adult patients with severe sepsis and septic shock: A meta-analysis of randomized clinical trials. Critical Care. 2014;**18**(6):702

[48] Rochwerg B, Alhazzani W, Gibson A, Ribic CM, Sindi A, Heels-Ansdell D, et al. Fluid type and the use of renal replacement therapy in sepsis: A systematic review and network meta-analysis. Intensive Care Medicine. 2015;**41**(9):1561-1571

[49] Caironi P, Tognoni G, Masson S, Fumagalli R, Pesenti A, Romero M, et al. Albumin replacement in patients with severe sepsis or septic shock. The New England Journal of Medicine. 2014;**370**(15):1412-1421

[50] Oliveira RP, Velasco I, Soriano FG, Friedman G. Clinical review: Hypertonic saline resuscitation in sepsis. Critical Care. 2002;**6**(5):418-423

[51] Li F, Sun H, Han XD. The effect of different fluids on early fluid resuscitation in septic shock. Zhongguo Wei Zhong Bing Ji Jiu Yi Xue. 2008;**20**(8):472-475

[52] Zhu GC, Quan ZY, Shao YS, Zhao JG, Zhang YT. The study of hypertonic saline and hydroxyethyl starch treating severe sepsis. Zhongguo Wei Zhong Bing Ji Jiu Yi Xue. 2011;**23**(3):150-153

[53] Raghunathan K, Bonavia A, Nathanson BH, Beadles CA, Shaw AD, Brookhart MA, et al. Association between initial fluid choice and subsequent in-hospital mortality during the resuscitation of adults with septic shock. Anesthesiology. 2015;**123**(6):1385-1393

[54] Chua HR, Venkatesh B, Stachowski E, Schneider AG, Perkins K, Ladanyi S, et al. Plasma-Lyte 148 vs 0.9% saline for fluid resuscitation in diabetic ketoacidosis. Journal of Critical Care. 2012;**27**(2):138-145

[55] Gosmanov AR, Gosmanova EO, Kitabchi AE. Hyperglycemic crises: Diabetic ketoacidosis (DKA), and hyperglycemic hyperosmolar state (HHS). In: De Groot LJ, Chrousos G, Dungan K, Feingold KR, Grossman A, Hershman JM, et al., editors. Endotext. South Dartmouth, MA: MDText.com, Inc.; 2000

[56] Kitabchi AE, Umpierrez GE, Miles JM, Fisher JN. Hyperglycemic crises in adult patients with diabetes. Diabetes Care. 2009;**32**(7):1335-1343

[57] Padhi S, Bullock I, Li L, Stroud M. National Institute for H, Care Excellence Guideline Development G. Intravenous fluid therapy for adults in hospital: Summary of NICE guidance. BMJ. 2013;**347**:f7073

[58] Corona G, Giuliani C, Parenti G, Norello D, Verbalis JG, Forti G, et al. Moderate hyponatremia is associated with increased risk of mortality: Evidence from a meta-analysis. PLoS One. 2013;**8**(12):e80451

[59] Upadhyay A, Jaber BL, Madias NE. Epidemiology of hyponatremia. Seminars in Nephrology. 2009;**29**(3):227-238

[60] Hawkins RC. Age and gender as risk factors for hyponatremia and hypernatremia. Clinica Chimica Acta. 2003;**337**(1-2):169-172

[61] Miller M, Hecker MS, Friedlander DA, Carter JM. Apparent idiopathic hyponatremia in an ambulatory geriatric population. Journal of the American Geriatrics Society. 1996; **44**(4):404-408

[62] Miller M, Morley JE, Rubenstein LZ. Hyponatremia in a nursing home population. Journal of the American Geriatrics Society. 1995;**43**(12):1410-1413

[63] Liamis G, Rodenburg EM, Hofman A, Zietse R, Stricker BH, Hoorn EJ. Electrolyte disorders in community subjects: Prevalence and risk factors. The American Journal of Medicine. 2013;**126**(3):256-263

[64] Verbalis JG, Goldsmith SR, Greenberg A, Korzelius C, Schrier RW, Sterns RH, et al. Diagnosis, evaluation, and treatment of hyponatremia: Expert panel recommendations. The American Journal of Medicine. 2013;**126**(10, Suppl 1):S1-S42

[65] Spasovski G, Vanholder R, Allolio B, Annane D, Ball S, Bichet D, et al. Clinical practice guideline on diagnosis and treatment of hyponatraemia. European Journal of Endocrinology. 2014;**170**(3):G1-G47

[66] Spasovski G, Vanholder R, Allolio B, Annane D, Ball S, Bichet D, et al. Clinical practice guideline on diagnosis and treatment of hyponatraemia. Nephrology, Dialysis, Transplantation. 2014;**29**(Suppl 2):i1-i39

[67] Spasovski G, Vanholder R, Allolio B, Annane D, Ball S, Bichet D, et al. Clinical practice guideline on diagnosis and treatment of hyponatraemia. Intensive Care Medicine. 2014; **40**(3):320-331

[68] Halperin ML, Kamel KS. Fluid, Electrolyte, and Acid-base Physiology: A Problem-based Approach. Philadelphia, PA: Elsevier; 2017. Available from: EBSCOhost http://search.ebscohost.com/login.aspx?direct=true&scope=site&db=nlebk&db=nlabk&AN=1389309; ScienceDirect http://www.sciencedirect.com/science/book/9780323355155 R2 Digital Library http://www.r2library.com/Resource/Title/0323355153; http://0-www.sciencedirect.com.pugwash.lib.warwick.ac.uk/science/book/9780323355155; http://libproxy.cbu.ca:2048/login?url=http://search.ebscohost.com/login.aspx?direct=true&db=nlebk&AN=1389309&site=ehost-live&scope=site

[69] Wald R, Jaber BL, Price LL, Upadhyay A, Madias NE. Impact of hospital-associated hyponatremia on selected outcomes. Archives of Internal Medicine. 2010;**170**(3):294-302

[70] Kim GH. Pseudohyponatremia: Does it matter in current clinical practice? Electrolyte & Blood Pressure: E & BP. 2006;**4**(2):77-82

[71] Fisher PG. 50 years ago in the Journal of Pediatrics: Cerebrospinal fluid and blood electrolytes in 62 mentally defective infants and children. The Journal of Pediatrics. 2014;**165**(3):515

[72] Hoorn EJ, Zietse R. Diagnosis and treatment of hyponatremia: Compilation of the guidelines. Journal of the American Society of Nephrology. 2017;**28**(5):1340-1349

[73] Chung HM, Kluge R, Schrier RW, Anderson RJ. Clinical assessment of extracellular fluid volume in hyponatremia. The American Journal of Medicine. 1987;**83**(5):905-908

[74] McGee S, Abernethy WB 3rd, Simel DL. The rational clinical examination. Is this patient hypovolemic? Journal of the American Medical Association. 1999;**281**(11):1022-1029

[75] Musch W, Thimpont J, Vandervelde D, Verhaeverbeke I, Berghmans T, Decaux G. Combined fractional excretion of sodium and urea better predicts response to saline in hyponatremia than do usual clinical and biochemical parameters. The American Journal of Medicine. 1995;**99**(4):348-355

[76] Hoorn EJ, Halperin ML, Zietse R. Diagnostic approach to a patient with hyponatraemia: Traditional versus physiology-based options. QJM. 2005;**98**(7):529-540

[77] Tasdemir V, Oguz AK, Sayin I, Ergun I. Hyponatremia in the outpatient setting: Clinical characteristics, risk factors, and outcome. International Urology and Nephrology. 2015;**47**(12):1977-1983

[78] Kengne FG, Decaux G. CNS manifestations of hyponatremia and its treatment. In: Simon EE, editor. Hyponatremia: Evaluation and Treatment. New York, NY: Springer New York; 2013. pp. 87-110

[79] Babaliche P, Madnani S, Kamat S. Clinical profile of patients admitted with hyponatremia in the medical intensive care unit. Indian Journal of Critical Care Medicine. 2017;**21**(12):819-824

[80] Nagler EV, Vanmassenhove J, van der Veer SN, Nistor I, Van Biesen W, Webster AC, et al. Diagnosis and treatment of hyponatremia: A systematic review of clinical practice guidelines and consensus statements. BMC Medicine. 2014;**12**:1

[81] Hoorn EJ, Hotho D, Hassing RJ, Zietse R. Unexplained hyponatremia: Seek and you will find. Nephron. Physiology. 2011;**118**(3):p66-p71

[82] Roussel R, Fezeu L, Marre M, Velho G, Fumeron F, Jungers P, et al. Comparison between copeptin and vasopressin in a population from the community and in people with chronic kidney disease. The Journal of Clinical Endocrinology and Metabolism. 2014;**99**(12):4656-4663

[83] Moses AM, Clayton B. Impairment of osmotically stimulated AVP release in patients with primary polydipsia. The American Journal of Physiology. 1993;**265**(6 Pt 2):R1247-R1252

[84] Fenske W, Stork S, Blechschmidt A, Maier SG, Morgenthaler NG, Allolio B. Copeptin in the differential diagnosis of hyponatremia. The Journal of Clinical Endocrinology and Metabolism. 2009;**94**(1):123-129

[85] Blanchard A, Steichen O, De Mota N, Curis E, Gauci C, Frank M, et al. An abnormal apelin/vasopressin balance may contribute to water retention in patients with the syndrome of inappropriate antidiuretic hormone (SIADH) and heart failure. The Journal of Clinical Endocrinology and Metabolism. 2013;**98**(5):2084-2089

[86] Nigro N, Winzeler B, Suter-Widmer I, Schuetz P, Arici B, Bally M, et al. Mid-regional pro-atrial natriuretic peptide and the assessment of volaemic status and differential diagnosis of profound hyponatraemia. Journal of Internal Medicine. 2015;**278**(1):29-37

[87] Hus-Citharel A, Bodineau L, Frugiere A, Joubert F, Bouby N, Llorens-Cortes C. Apelin counteracts vasopressin-induced water reabsorption via cross talk between apelin and vasopressin receptor signaling pathways in the rat collecting duct. Endocrinology. 2014;**155**(11):4483-4493

[88] Tzikas S, Keller T, Wild PS, Schulz A, Zwiener I, Zeller T, et al. Midregional pro-atrial natriuretic peptide in the general population/Insights from the Gutenberg Health Study. Clinical Chemistry and Laboratory Medicine. 2013;**51**(5):1125-1133

[89] Hoorn EJ, Lindemans J, Zietse R. Development of severe hyponatraemia in hospitalized patients: Treatment-related risk factors and inadequate management. Nephrology, Dialysis, Transplantation. 2006;**21**(1):70-76

[90] Cohen DM, Ellison DH. Evaluating hyponatremia. Journal of the American Medical Association. 2015;**313**(12):1260-1261

[91] Moritz ML, Ayus JC. The syndrome of inappropriate antidiuresis. The New England Journal of Medicine. 2007;**357**(9):942 author reply

[92] Musch W, Decaux G. Treating the syndrome of inappropriate ADH secretion with isotonic saline. QJM. 1998;**91**(11):749-753

[93] Steele A, Gowrishankar M, Abrahamson S, Mazer CD, Feldman RD, Halperin ML. Postoperative hyponatremia despite near-isotonic saline infusion: A phenomenon of desalination. Annals of Internal Medicine. 1997;**126**(1):20-25

[94] Hauptman PJ, Burnett J, Gheorghiade M, Grinfeld L, Konstam MA, Kostic D, et al. Clinical course of patients with hyponatremia and decompensated systolic heart failure and the effect of vasopressin receptor antagonism with tolvaptan. Journal of Cardiac Failure. 2013;**19**(6):390-397

[95] Konstam MA, Gheorghiade M, Burnett JC Jr, Grinfeld L, Maggioni AP, Swedberg K, et al. Effects of oral tolvaptan in patients hospitalized for worsening heart failure: The EVEREST Outcome Trial. Journal of the American Medical Association. 2007; **297**(12):1319-1331

[96] Ayus JC, Armstrong D, Arieff AI. Hyponatremia with hypoxia: Effects on brain adaptation, perfusion, and histology in rodents. Kidney International. 2006;**69**(8):1319-1325

[97] Ayus JC, Arieff AI. Pulmonary complications of hyponatremic encephalopathy. Noncardiogenic pulmonary edema and hypercapnic respiratory failure. Chest. 1995; **107**(2):517-521

[98] Huq S, Wong M, Chan H, Crimmins D. Osmotic demyelination syndromes: Central and extrapontine myelinolysis. Journal of Clinical Neuroscience. 2007;**14**(7):684-688

[99] Berl T. Vasopressin antagonists. The New England Journal of Medicine. 2015;**372**(23): 2207-2216

[100] Lehrich RW, Ortiz-Melo DI, Patel MB, Greenberg A. Role of vaptans in the management of hyponatremia. American Journal of Kidney Diseases. 2013;**62**(2):364-376

[101] Berl T, Quittnat-Pelletier F, Verbalis JG, Schrier RW, Bichet DG, Ouyang J, et al. Oral tolvaptan is safe and effective in chronic hyponatremia. Journal of the American Society of Nephrology. 2010;**21**(4):705-712

[102] Schrier RW, Gross P, Gheorghiade M, Berl T, Verbalis JG, Czerwiec FS, et al. Tolvaptan, a selective oral vasopressin V2-receptor antagonist, for hyponatremia. The New England Journal of Medicine. 2006;**355**(20):2099112

[103] Tzoulis P, Waung JA, Bagkeris E, Carr H, Khoo B, Cohen M, et al. Real-life experience of tolvaptan use in the treatment of severe hyponatraemia due to syndrome of inappropriate antidiuretic hormone secretion. Clinical Endocrinology. 2016;**84**(4):620-626

[104] Sarges P, Steinberg JM, Lewis JH. Drug-induced liver injury: Highlights from a review of the 2015 literature. Drug Safety. 2016;**39**(9):801-821

[105] Dousa TP, Wilson DM. Effects of demethylchlortetracycline on cellular action of antidiuretic hormone in vitro. Kidney International. 1974;**5**(4):279-284

[106] Kruse C, Eiken P, Verbalis J, Vestergaard P. The effect of chronic mild hyponatremia on bone mineral loss evaluated by retrospective national Danish patient data. Bone. 2016;**84**:9-14

[107] Usala RL, Fernandez SJ, Mete M, Cowen L, Shara NM, Barsony J, et al. Hyponatremia is associated with increased osteoporosis and bone fractures in a large US health system population. The Journal of Clinical Endocrinology and Metabolism. 2015; **100**(8):3021-3031

[108] Holm JP, Amar AOS, Hyldstrup L, Jensen JEB. Hyponatremia, a risk factor for osteoporosis and fractures in women. Osteoporosis International. 2016;**27**(3):989-1001

[109] Kwak MK, Choi D, Lee JH, Kim HJ, Park HK, Suh KI, et al. Relationship between decrease in serum sodium level and bone mineral density in osteoporotic fracture patients. Journal of Bone Metabolism. 2015;**22**(1):915

[110] Kruse C, Eiken P, Vestergaard P. Hyponatremia and osteoporosis: Insights from the Danish National Patient Registry. Osteoporosis International. 2015;**26**(3):1005-1016

[111] Kinsella S, Moran S, Sullivan MO, Molloy MG, Eustace JA. Hyponatremia independent of osteoporosis is associated with fracture occurrence. Clinical Journal of the American Society of Nephrology. 2010;**5**(2):275-280

[112] Melton JE, Nattie EE. Brain and CSF water and ions during dilutional and isosmotic hyponatremia in the rat. The American Journal of Physiology. 1983;**244**(5):R724-R732

[113] Verbalis JG, Drutarosky MD. Adaptation to chronic hypoosmolality in rats. Kidney International. 1988;**34**(3):351-360

[114] Verbalis JG, Gullans SR. Hyponatremia causes large sustained reductions in brain content of multiple organic osmolytes in rats. Brain Research. 1991;**567**(2):274-282

[115] Videen JS, Michaelis T, Pinto P, Ross BD. Human cerebral osmolytes during chronic hyponatremia. A proton magnetic resonance spectroscopy study. The Journal of Clinical Investigation. 1995;**95**(2):788-793

[116] Arieff AI. Hyponatremia, convulsions, respiratory arrest, and permanent brain damage after elective surgery in healthy women. The New England Journal of Medicine. 1986;**314**(24):1529-1535

[117] Arieff AI, Llach F, Massry SG. Neurological manifestations and morbidity of hyponatremia: Correlation with brain water and electrolytes. Medicine (Baltimore). 1976; **55**(2):121-129

[118] Ayus JC, Krothapalli RK, Arieff AI. Treatment of symptomatic hyponatremia and its relation to brain damage. A prospective study. The New England Journal of Medicine. 1987;**317**(19):1190-1195

[119] Gankam-Kengne F, Ayers C, Khera A, de Lemos J, Maalouf NM. Mild hyponatremia is associated with an increased risk of death in an ambulatory setting. Kidney International. 2013;**83**(4):700-706

[120] Mohan S, Gu S, Parikh A, Radhakrishnan J. Prevalence of hyponatremia and association with mortality: Results from NHANES. The American Journal of Medicine. 2013;**126**(12):1127-1137 e1

[121] Rusinaru D, Tribouilloy C, Berry C, Richards AM, Whalley GA, Earle N, et al. Relationship of serum sodium concentration to mortality in a wide spectrum of heart failure patients with preserved and with reduced ejection fraction: An individual patient data meta-analysis(dagger): Meta-Analysis Global Group in Chronic heart failure (MAGGIC). European Journal of Heart Failure. 2012;**14**(10):1139-1146

[122] Gheorghiade M, Abraham WT, Albert NM, Gattis Stough W, Greenberg BH, O'Connor CM, et al. Relationship between admission serum sodium concentration and clinical outcomes in patients hospitalized for heart failure: An analysis from the OPTIMIZE-HF registry. European Heart Journal. 2007;**28**(8):980-988

[123] Shorr AF, Tabak YP, Johannes RS, Gupta V, Saltzberg MT, Costanzo MR. Burden of sodium abnormalities in patients hospitalized for heart failure. Congestive Heart Failure. 2011;**17**(1):1-7

[124] Kim WR, Biggins SW, Kremers WK, Wiesner RH, Kamath PS, Benson JT, et al. Hyponatremia and mortality among patients on the liver-transplant waiting list. The New England Journal of Medicine. 2008;**359**(10):1018-1026

[125] Kovesdy CP, Lott EH, Lu JL, Malakauskas SM, Ma JZ, Molnar MZ, et al. Hyponatremia, hypernatremia, and mortality in patients with chronic kidney disease with and without congestive heart failure. Circulation. 2012;**125**(5):677-684

[126] Nigwekar SU, Wenger J, Thadhani R, Bhan I. Hyponatremia, mineral metabolism, and mortality in incident maintenance hemodialysis patients: A cohort study. American Journal of Kidney Diseases. 2013;**62**(4):755-762

[127] Chang TI, Kim YL, Kim H, Ryu GW, Kang EW, Park JT, et al. Hyponatremia as a predictor of mortality in peritoneal dialysis patients. PLoS One. 2014;**9**(10):e111373

[128] Zilberberg MD, Exuzides A, Spalding J, Foreman A, Jones AG, Colby C, et al. Hyponatremia and hospital outcomes among patients with pneumonia: A retrospective cohort study. BMC Pulmonary Medicine. 2008;**8**:16

[129] Tang WW, Kaptein EM, Feinstein EI, Massry SG. Hyponatremia in hospitalized patients with the acquired immunodeficiency syndrome (AIDS) and the AIDS-related complex. The American Journal of Medicine. 1993;**94**(2):16974

[130] Tamizifar B, Kheiry S, Fereidoony F. Hyponatremia and 30 days mortality of patients with acute pulmonary embolism. Journal of Research in Medical Sciences. 2015; **20**(8):777-781

[131] Scherz N, Labarere J, Mean M, Ibrahim SA, Fine MJ, Aujesky D. Prognostic importance of hyponatremia in patients with acute pulmonary embolism. American Journal of Respiratory and Critical Care Medicine. 2010;**182**(9):1178-1183

[132] Waikar SS, Mount DB, Curhan GC. Mortality after hospitalization with mild, moderate, and severe hyponatremia. The American Journal of Medicine. 2009;**122**(9):857-865

[133] Vandergheynst F, Gombeir Y, Bellante F, Perrotta G, Remiche G, Melot C, et al. Impact of hyponatremia on nerve conduction and muscle strength. European Journal of Clinical Investigation. 2016;**46**(4):328-333

[134] Renneboog B, Musch W, Vandemergel X, Manto MU, Decaux G. Mild chronic hyponatremia is associated with falls, unsteadiness, and attention deficits. The American Journal of Medicine. 2006;**119**(1):71 e1-71 e8

[135] de Souza A, Desai PK. More often striatal myelinolysis than pontine? A consecutive series of patients with osmotic demyelination syndrome. Neurological Research. 2012; **34**(3):262-271

[136] Sterns RH, Riggs JE, Schochet SS Jr. Osmotic demyelination syndrome following correction of hyponatremia. The New England Journal of Medicine. 1986;**314**(24):1535-1542

[137] Menger H, Jorg J. Outcome of central pontine and extrapontine myelinolysis (n = 44). Journal of Neurology. 1999;**246**(8):700-705

[138] Louis G, Megarbane B, Lavoue S, Lassalle V, Argaud L, Poussel JF, et al. Long-term outcome of patients hospitalized in intensive care units with central or extrapontine myelinolysis. Critical Care Medicine. 2012;**40**(3):970-972

[139] Kallakatta RN, Radhakrishnan A, Fayaz RK, Unnikrishnan JP, Kesavadas C, Sarma SP. Clinical and functional outcome and factors predicting prognosis in osmotic demyelination syndrome (central pontine and/or extrapontine myelinolysis) in 25 patients. Journal of Neurology, Neurosurgery, and Psychiatry. 2011;**82**(3):326-331

[140] Sood L, Sterns RH, Hix JK, Silver SM, Chen L. Hypertonic saline and desmopressin: A simple strategy for safe correction of severe hyponatremia. American Journal of Kidney Diseases. 2013;**61**(4):571-578

[141] Perianayagam A, Sterns RH, Silver SM, Grieff M, Mayo R, Hix J, et al. DDAVP is effective in preventing and reversing inadvertent overcorrection of hyponatremia. Clinical Journal of the American Society of Nephrology. 2008;**3**(2):331-336

[142] Soupart A, Penninckx R, Crenier L, Stenuit A, Perier O, Decaux G. Prevention of brain demyelination in rats after excessive correction of chronic hyponatremia by serum sodium lowering. Kidney International. 1994;**45**(1):193-200

[143] Gankam Kengne F, Soupart A, Pochet R, Brion JP, Decaux G. Re-induction of hyponatremia after rapid overcorrection of hyponatremia reduces mortality in rats. Kidney International. 2009;**76**(6):614-621

[144] Adrogue HJ, Madias NE. Hypernatremia. The New England Journal of Medicine. 2000;**342**(20):1493-1499

[145] Liamis G, Filippatos TD, Elisaf MS. Evaluation and treatment of hypernatremia: A practical guide for physicians. Postgraduate Medicine. 2016;**128**(3):299-306

[146] Sterns RH. Disorders of plasma sodium—Causes, consequences, and correction. The New England Journal of Medicine. 2015;**372**(1):55-65

Chapter 2

Hyponatremia and Psychotropic Drugs

Mireia Martínez Cortés and Pedro Gurillo Muñoz

Additional information is available at the end of the chapter

http://dx.doi.org/10.5772/intechopen.79029

Abstract

Given the widespread use of psychotropic drugs in the population, it's important to consider hyponatremia as an avoidable and reversible adverse effect and include the detection of high-risk subjects to establish safer medications, as well as early detection measures in routine clinical practice. Although hyponatremia has been especially associated with serotonergic antidepressants (SSRIs), there is also an elevated risk with tricyclics, duals and heterocyclic antidepressants, due to the different mechanisms of action at the renal tubular level and the release of ADH. Hyponatremia secondary to tricyclics with slow CYP2D6 metabolizers have higher plasma concentrations of antidepressants metabolized by CYP2D6. Hyponatremia secondary to SSRIs appears in the first week of treatment, it is "not dose-dependent" and normalization of natremia occurs between 2 and 20 days after stopping the medication. Bupropion, trazodone, mianserin, reboxetine and agomelatine are a safe alternative. Also antiepileptics have been related to hyponatremia. Both typical and atypical antipsychotics have been exposed to an increased risk of hyponatremia, even after adjusted factors such as age, sex and comorbidity. Other factors that favor the onset of hyponatremia act synergistically with psychotropic drugs, such as: advanced age, female sex, concomitant diuretic intake, low body weight and low sodium levels; NSAID, ACEIs, and warm.

Keywords: hyponatremia, antipsychotic, antidepressant, antiepileptic, psychotropic drugs

1. Introduction

Hyponatremia is the most frequent hydroelectrolytic disorder in clinical practice, both in hospital and outpatient settings [1]. Defined as a serum sodium concentration or sodium level < 135 mmol/L, its frequency varies according to its intensity, with severe and more severe hyponatremia in hospitalized patients. Hyponatremia is present in 15–20% of urgent hospital admissions and in up to 20% of critical patients. Although it estimates a daily incidence of 1% in hospitalized patients and a prevalence of 2.5%, its frequency is probably higher, since it is frequently underdiagnosed [2]. Some epidemiological studies report that only 30% of patients with hyponatremia are diagnosed, including the most serious ones [3]. Clinical manifestations of hyponatremia have a broad spectrum, from mild to severe or even potentially lethal. Hyponatremia is related to an increase in mortality, morbidity, duration of hospital stay and socio-health costs in patients with multiple pathologies. Some studies show that the presence of hyponatremia is an independent predictor of mortality rate, implying a relative risk of death between 1 and 2 times higher [4]; risk that is maintained per year and even 5 years after a hospital admission. Hyponatremia is related to a higher rate of hospitalization in Intensive Care Units and mechanical ventilation units.

Etiology of hyponatremia is multifactorial, highlighting the pharmacological origin. Some of the mechanisms involved in the development of pharmacological hyponatremia are the alteration of sodium and water homeostasis (diuretics), the increase in the production of the antidiuretic hormone (antidepressants, antipsychotics, antiepileptics, anticancer drugs, methrotrexate, interferon alfa, opiates) and the potentiation of the effects of antidiuretic hormone (antiepileptic, hypoglycemic, nonsteroidal anti-inflammatory drugs [NSAIDs], angiotensin-converting enzyme inhibitors [ACEIs] and anticancer drugs). Factors such as female sex, weight, advanced age, the presence of associated pathologies (cardiological, hepatic, neurological and endocrine), the concomitant use of drugs (especially thiazide diuretics, inhibitors of the reuptake of serotonin and carbamazepine) and basal sodium levels in the low threshold of normality have been related to the development of hyponatremia [5].

Prescription and use of psychotropic drugs is currently growing, both due to the increase in the incidence of mental illnesses and depression, which according to the WHO will be the second cause of disability in the world in 2020 [6]. Elderly patients have higher prevalences of mood disorders, which together with the greater frequency of polypathology and polypharmacy, makes them a risk group for presenting hyponatremia.

2. Hyponatremia

2.1. Definition of hyponatremia

2.1.1. Definition of hyponatremia based on biochemical severity

Mild (sodium between 130 and 135 mmol/L); moderate (sodium between 125 and 129 mmol/L); severe (sodium <125 mmol/L).

2.1.2. Definition of hyponatremia based on development time

Acute (<48 h) or chronic (greater or equal to 48 h). Current literature establishes the limit of 48 h to distinguish between acute and chronic hyponatremia, since cerebral edema appears more frequently when hyponatremia is established in less than 48 h. Experimental studies suggest that the brain needs approximately 48 h to adapt to a hypotonic environment; there is a risk of cerebral edema before such adaptation. However, once the adaptation is completed, a rapid rise in the serum sodium level can cause lesions of the myelin sheath, which is known as osmotic demyelination syndrome. Hence, the importance in clinical practice to distinguish between acute and chronic hyponatremia, evaluating whether a subject is at greater risk of cerebral edema or osmotic demyelination. If there are doubts about the development time of hyponatremia [7], it should be considered chronic, unless there are reasons to think otherwise.

2.1.3. Definition of hyponatremia based on symptoms

Moderate: any degree of hyponatremia associated with moderately severe symptoms of hyponatremia: nausea without vomiting, confusion, and headache.

Severe: any biochemical degree of hyponatremia associated with severe symptoms of hyponatremia: vomiting, cardiorespiratory distress, abnormal and deep drowsiness, seizures, and coma.

2.1.4. Definition of hyponatremia based on plasma osmolality

- **Hypotonic hyponatremia:** the decrease in extracellular sodium is accompanied by hypotonia of the extracellular fluid and displacement of water from the extracellular space to the intracellular space, causing cellular edema. The most frequent cause is a syndrome of inappropriate secretion of antidiuretic hormone (SIADH). There are three types according to the volume status:

    a. *hypotonic hyponatremia with hypovolemia*: occurs when there are losses of sodium and water, with partial supplementation of fluid losses without electrolytes. Losses can occur through the skin, digestive tract, renal pathway or leakage of fluids into a third space.

    b. *hypotonic hyponatremia with isovolemia*: SIADH is the most common cause of hyponatremia.

    c. *hypotonic hyponatremia with hypervolemia*: it occurs both in situations of increased vasopressin secretion in states of a relative decrease in effective intravascular volume (chronic heart failure, liver cirrhosis with ascites, nephrotic edema); excessive fluid intake without electrolytes and an altered excretion of free water (acute kidney injury, advanced chronic kidney disease).

- **Nonhypotonic hyponatremia (isotonic or hypertonic):** increase in the plasma concentration of effective osmoles displaces the water from the intracellular to the extracellular space and generates a dilutional hyponatremia. Depending on the concentration of these compounds the plasma osmolality may be normal or increased. The most frequent cause is hyperglycemia.

- **Fictional hyponatremia or pseudohyponatremia** occurs when a plasma concentration of sodium falsely decreases as a result of a high concentration of lipids or paraproteins, with normal plasma osmolality.

2.2. Etiology

2.2.1. Acute hyponatremia

Primary polydipsia, intensive physical exercise, thiazide diuretics, postoperative state, vasopressin analogs, colonoscopy preparations, 3,4-methylenedioxymethamphetamine intake.

2.2.2. Nonhypotonic hyponatremia

- *Isotonic or hypertonic*: secondary to the presence of effective osmoles (glucose, mannitol, glycine, hyperosmolar radiological contrast, maltose).
- *Isotonic or hyperosmolar:* secondary to presence of ineffective osmoles that elevate measured serum osmolality but do not cause hyponatremia because they do not change effective osmolality and does not attract water to extracellular compartment (urea, alcohol).
- *Isotonic:* presence of endogenous solutes that cause pseudohyponatremia (triglycerides, cholesterol, proteins, intravenous immunoglobulins, monoclonal gammopathies).

2.2.3. Hypotonic hyponatremia

- *Hypovolemic*: excessive sweating, vomiting, diarrhea, digestive tract fistulas, diuretics, tubulopathies, mineralocorticoid deficiency.
- *Hypervolemic*: chronic heart failure, liver cirrhosis, nephrotic edema, ascites, acute and chronic renal failure.
- *Isovolemia*: syndrome of inappropriate secretion of antidiuretic hormone (SIADH) which can be secondary to tumors (lung, oropharynx, stomach, duodenum, pancreas, ureter, bladder, prostate, endometrium, Ewing sarcoma, lymphomas, neuroblastoma), nervous system disorder (encephalitis, meningitis, abscess, infection by Rickettsia and Plasmodium, HIV, subdural hemorrhage, stroke, hydrocephalus, multiple sclerosis, Guillain-Barré syndrome, delirium tremens, acute porphyria), drugs (antidepressants, anticonvulsants, antipsychotics, anticancer drugs, antidiabetics, vasopressin analogs, opioids, interferon, NSAIDs, clofibrate, nicotine, proton pump inhibitors, amiodarone) [7].

2.2.4. Hyponatremia and psychotropic drugs

As we have previously described, in case of psychotropic drugs, hyponatremia is mediated by the inappropriate release of ADH. ADH or vasopressin is a hypothalamic hormone that is stored and released through the neurohypophysis in response to osmotic and nonosmotic stimuli:

1. Osmotic stimulus: the ADH is released or inhibited depending on the concentration of effective osmoles in the extracellular compartment. Osmotic threshold for ADH release is 280 – 290 mOsm/kg.
2. Nonosmotic stimulus:

- Hemodynamics. In the presence of low effective circulating volume, the baroreceptors are activated. For example: hypovolemia, liver cirrhosis, arterial hypotension, congestive heart failure, nephrotic syndrome, primary adrenal insufficiency.
- Nonhemodynamic: mediated by the release of corticotropin-releasing hormone (CRH, neurotransmitter involved in the response to stress and responsible for activating the pituitary secretion of ACTH) and angiotensin II. For example: pain, stress, nausea and vomiting, hypoglycemia, drugs, cancer, postoperative state, pulmonary or central nervous system pathology.

Vasopressin has three receptors coupled to G proteins: V1 (presents vasopressor effect), V2 (responsible for the reabsorption of water in the collecting tubule of the nephron) and V3 (responsible for the release of ACTH). Vasopressin or ADH has several functions:

1. Renal. ADH acts on V2 receptors on collecting duct in the nephron. Its action increases the reabsorption of water, but not of solute, through the increased expression of aquaporin 2 channels (AQP2). Aquaporins are proteins that are part of the water channel. AQP2 is expressed exclusively in collecting duct principal cells and is responsible for the apical water permeability of this region of the nephron. Its activity is dependent on ADH, which is released in response to hyperosmolar and hypovolemic stimuli. There is a type of inherited nephrogenic diabetes insipidus associated with mutations in AQP2 [8].
2. Vascular smooth muscle. It produces vasoconstriction and increases peripheral vascular resistance.

2.3. Symptomatology

The symptomatology of hyponatremia varies depending on the biochemical severity and the speed of the establishment. It can be classified as mild, moderate and severe.

2.3.1. Mild symptoms

(Na 130–135 mEq/L): headache, attention deficit, memory alterations, irritability, depression.

2.3.2. Moderate symptoms

(Na 120–130 mEq/L): nausea, vomiting, bradypsychia, confusion, disorientation.

2.3.3. Severe symptoms

(Na < 120 mEq/L): stupor, seizures, coma, respiratory depression.

2.3.4. Hyponatremic encephalopathy

In hyponatremia, low serum osmolarity causes an osmotic gradient between the extracellular space and the intracellular space, with the consequent passage of free water into the interior of the cell. This accumulation of water in the brain cells causes cerebral edema. The cellular edema produces an increase in the size of the various organs, however in the case of brain, expansion is not possible due to the limitation of the cranial cavity. Thus, increases in brain volume of 8–10% can cause coma and compromise the condition of the individual due to intracranial hypertension and transtentorial herniation. However, hyponatremia activates a series of compensatory mechanisms to decrease the volume of intracellular fluid, to reduce the risk of cerebral edema and the risks derived from it [9]. Adequate regulation of brain volume is an essential factor in the prognosis of hyponatremic encephalopathy. Some of these compensatory mechanisms are:

1. The increase in intracranial pressure favors the increase of hydrostatic pressure and subsequent passage of water to the ventricular and venous system.
2. After an initial osmotic edema, the cells quickly expel electrolytes (potassium, chloride and sodium) into the extracellular space, with the subsequent release of water by osmotic gradient, restoring brain volume. This phenomenon allows to restore cell volume in hours but is energy dependent and requires the operation of sodium-potassium ATPase system.
3. Role of the astrocytes. Act as regulators of brain water content, its swelling in hyposmolar situations protect and spare neurons. Its extensions form the blood-brain barrier and they have high number of pores called aquaporins (AQP) particularly AQP1 and AQP4, allowing the passage of water into astrocytes in hyposmolar situations which selectively swell, whereas neurons are relatively spared.
4. Studies in animals have shown that brain osmolytes (glycine, taurine, creatine myo-inositol) leave the cell in hypoosmolar states and accumulate in the hyperosmolar states. Studies in humans with magnetic resonance imaging show that the osmolytes output is parallel to the changes in sodium concentration, which takes approximately 48 h.

Brain adaptation to hyponatremia is related to the speed of its establishment. In chronic hyponatremia (that lasts more than 48 h) the slow and progressive decrease of sodium allows a compensatory regulation of the whole volume, limiting the degree of cerebral edema and being asymptomatic or slightly symptomatic. However, in cases of acute hyponatremia, adaptive mechanisms are exceeded and symptoms are more likely to occur even with mild hyponatremia.

There are some risk factors for the development of hyponatremic cerebral edema:

- Menstruating women. Estrogens inhibit the sodium-potassium ATPase, making intracellular sodium leakage difficult; and affect the expression of AQP4 channels. In this patient profile, cases of hyponatremic encephalopathy with cerebral herniation have been documented even with serum sodium of 128 mEq/L.
- Children. They are a risk group for unfavorable evolution in hyponatremic encephalopathy. It is postulated that the high ratio of brain size to that of the skull after the closure of the fontanelles, as well as the lower activity of the sodium-potassium ATPase pump than in adults can limit the adaptation to cerebral edema.

- Hypoxia It has been postulated that hypoxia is a factor for death and brain damage in patients with hyponatremia, after adjustment for other comorbidities. It alters the regulation of the energy-dependent astrocyte volume, since the active transport of sodium requires oxygen. In addition, in patients with hyponatremic encephalopathy, cranial hypertension and incipient brain herniation may favor the development of a neurogenic pulmonary edema and hypercapnic respiratory failure that worsens hypoxia.
- Hormonal factors: vasopressin and estrogen make it difficult to adapt to cellular edema. On the one hand, vasopressin acts by decreasing brain flow and oxygen consumption through arterial vasoconstriction, as well as facilitating the displacement of water in brain cells through AQP4. On the other hand, estrogens increase the secretion of vasopressin.
- Risk factors to develop hyponatremia: as we have previously commented, the establishment of the hyponatremia and the severity of it is associated with multiple factors such as polypathology and polymedication, among others. For this reason, literature recommends the identification of those risk factors to perform an adequate prevention and early detection of those cases of hyponatremia.

2.3.5. *Age*

Elderly patients are a vulnerable population and at risk of developing hyponatremia due to various causes. In the first place, the physiological changes characteristic of aging, such as the decrease in volume and body weight, pose a risk to develop hyponatremia. On the other hand, they are a population often with multi co-morbidities, exposed to diets without salt, to forced hydration (oral or intravenous) and with the use of polytherapy, which makes them candidates for risk.

2.3.6. *Institutionalization*

Some studies have shown a higher incidence of hyponatremia in subjects older than 60 years institutionalized in residences than in patients of the same age living at home (18 versus 8%) [10].

2.3.7. *Female sex*

Female sex has been associated with an increased risk of hyponatremia and the development of hyponatremic encephalopathy [11]. Some hypothesis proposed for this difference are based on hormonal factors and cellular transport of sodium and volume of distribution of body water different from men.

2.3.8. *Comorbidity*

Hyponatremia has been associated with multiple pathologies (infectious, oncological, neurological, renal, metabolic, etc.).

2.3.9. *Polytherapy*

Multiple drugs have been associated with an increased risk of hyponatremia, especially antipsychotics, antidepressants and antiepileptic [12], diuretics (mainly thiazides), ACEIs and NSAIDs. Other drugs have been related to hyponatremia, such as vasopressin analogs, interferon, antidiabetics, anticancer drugs, proton pump inhibitors and monoclonal antibodies, among others.

1. Basal levels of sodium in low range of normality
2. Low weight
3. Exposure to high temperatures

2.4. Treatment

It is important to remember that despite of the severity of the neurological signs and symptoms of acute hyponatremia, the correction of hyponatremia in a rapid and uncontrolled way can generate chronic neurological lesions due to osmotic demyelination. When there is a decrease in sodium, cells excrete organic solutes and other molecules to maintain homeostasis, in a process that can last between 48 and 72 h, so hyponatremia can be classified as acute or chronic if the duration is shorter or greater than 48 h, respectively.

It is recommended that sodium correction rate does not exceed 8 mmol/L in any 24-h period, being even lower in those patients susceptible to osmotic demyelination (as in the case of advanced cirrhosis, alcoholism or severe malnutrition). Even in patients with severe hyponatremia that are accompanied by severe neurological symptoms, 4 – 6 mEq/L rise in serum sodium is sufficient in the first 24-h (this target can be achieved in first few hours in severely symptomatic patients and then maintained at that level for the first 24-h). Three percent sodium chloride solution can be used to achieve this. It is important to remember that the recommended correction rates of 24 h should not be exceeded.

There is a series of formulas that allow to calculate in a quantitative way the effect of the prescribed fluid therapy on patient's serum sodium.

The **Adrogue-Madias Formula (AMF)** [13] helps to estimate the effect of a given fluid on serum sodium. It takes into account the sodium concentration and the total body weight (TBW) adjusted by a correction factor that varies according to age and sex. However, the AMF does not take into account the losses and the pathophysiology that underlies them and requires that sodium levels be monitored frequently during the infusion of the fluid.

Infusate formula: Adrogue-Madias formula.

$$\Delta[Na^+]_s = \frac{[Na^+ + K^+]_{inf} - [Na^+]_s}{TBW + 1} \quad (1)$$

However, this formula has the limitation of being approximate as rise in sodium level is often greater than that predicted by the formula.

Fluid restriction should be the first therapeutic measure in cases of euvolemic or hypervolemic hyponatremia. Depending on the severity of the hyponatremia and symptomatic severity, the fluid should be restricted to provide a negative fluid balance of approximately 500 ml per day.

There are several therapeutic options for the treatment of hyponatremia secondary to SIADH:

Demeclocycline. It is a tetracyclic antibiotic whose mechanism of action is the inhibition of ADH receptors in the renal distal tubule, inducing nephrogenic diabetes insipidus. It is administered in doses of (300 – 600 mg twice a day). Side effects include photosensitivity, nephrotoxicity and nausea.

Antagonists of the vasopressin receptor ("vaptans"). ADH or vasopressin acts at the level of various receptors: V1a (causes vasoconstriction), V1b (secretion of ACTH) and V2 (water reabsorption and release of von Willebrand factor and factor VIII). Drugs that act on V2 receptors at the tubular level increase the excretion of water (aquaresis).

- Tolvaptan: It has an action as a selective antagonist of the V2 receptors of vasopressin at the level of the renal tubule, increasing the free elimination of water. It has been used in patients with congestive heart failure, cirrhosis and SIADH. Although it has not shown a reduction in the rates of rehospitalization or death due to congestive heart failure, it improves sodium levels, fluid balance and symptoms of congestion. It is approved for the treatment of hypervolemic and euvolemic hyponatremia.
- Conivaptan: Antagonist of the V1a-V2 receptors with approval for the treatment of euvolemic and hypervolemic hyponatremia. Its use is limited to intravenous use at the hospital level.
- Lixivaptan: V2 receptor antagonist of vasopressin, used in euvolemic and hypervolemic hyponatremia.

3. Hyponatremia and antipsychotics

Antipsychotics are a family of drugs used primarily in the treatment of schizophrenia, bipolar disorder and other affective psychoses, but also in other neuropsychiatric disorders (such as dementia and autism), symptomatic treatment of acute confusional symptoms and other conditions not psychiatric (nausea, hiccups, migraine). Some studies show stability in the prevalence (2.05%) and incidence (0.66%) in the use of antipsychotics in the last decade, although showing an increase in its use in the infant-juvenile population and higher employment of second generation antipsychotics (SGAPs) [14]. Its mechanism of action is dopaminergic blocking. They are classified into two main groups: the classic or typical antipsychotics, which present a blockade of the D2 dopaminergic receptor and are effective in the positive symptoms of schizophrenia (hallucinations and delusions) but show extrapyramidal symptoms as the most notable side effects; and the atypical or second generation antipsychotics, in addition to blocking the D2 receptor, exhibit muscarinic, adrenergic, serotonergic and histamergic receptor activity, showing a broader spectrum of action (including positive and negative symptoms) and a different side effect profile of the typical ones (minor extrapyramidal symptoms, but weight gain, dry mouth, orthostatic hypotension, constipation, urinary retention, narrow-angle glaucoma, sedation).

Hyponatremia is an adverse effect described both in the case of classical and atypical antipsychotics. It is postulated that the etiopathogenesis of hyponatremia in atypical antipsychotics is mediated by the action of serotonin, both by the release of ADH induced by the stimulation of central receptors 5-HT2 and 5-HT1c and by the increase in the effects of ADH at the renal medullary level [15]. In the case of typical antipsychotics, prolonged blockade of dopamine D2 receptors stimulates the release of ADH and increases its peripheral response [16]. The occurrence of hyponatremia occurs in the first 3 weeks of treatment in up to 50% of cases, although cases have also been reported in patients undergoing long-term chronic treatments. On the other hand, in the case of antipsychotics, neither age nor female sex are risk factors. The chemical structure and receptor affinity profiles of the dopamine D2 receptor and serotonin 5-HT2A have not shown a variation with respect to the risk of hyponatremia [17]. Several studies describe that hyponatremia at admission is associated with greater medical deterioration in hospitalized psychiatric patients [18], therefore adequate clinical monitoring should be performed to identify and treat somatic pathologies and concomitant use of drugs. Also, it is recommended to measure serum sodium in those patients on antipsychotic treatment who present with seizures.

In a follow-up study over 15 years with a sample of 2051 patients diagnosed with schizophrenia [19] from 1998 to 2013, an incidence of hyponatremia of 6.7% was observed. The study showed that the use of antipsychotics, both typical and atypical, was associated with an elevated risk of hyponatremia with respect to the nonuse of antipsychotics, even after adjusting for age, sex and physical comorbidity. Age of diagnosis of the disease, low income, physical comorbidity, psychiatric admissions and concomitant treatment with carbamazepine were also associated with an increased risk of hyponatremia. Another retrospective study showed that treatment with atypical antipsychotics in the elderly was associated with a modest but statistically significant increase in the risk of hospitalization for hyponatremia in 30 days, an association that was smaller than other psychotropic drugs [20]. A systematic review on hyponatremia and the use of antipsychotics, published in 2010 [16], which includes 4 studies and 91 cases and series of cases, showed that the diagnosis of schizophrenia and male sex were more frequently associated with hyponatremia. Using the Naranjo Scale of Adverse Drug Reaction Probability Scale, in 80% of the cases possible causality was determined, in 19% probable causality and in 1% impossible causality. No significant association was found between daily doses of drugs and serum sodium or time to onset of hyponatremia. Currently, tolvaptan is positioned as a drug approved by the FDA in the treatment of euvolemic and hypervolemic hyponatremia, and useful in the management of hyponatremia associated with the use of antipsychotics [21].

3.1. First generation antipsychotics (FGAS)

In recent decades the use of typical antipsychotics has been progressively replaced by atypical ones, by the receptor profile and side effects. Nonetheless, haloperidol continues to be the drug of choice in the management of agitation and acute confusional syndrome. Haloperidol-related hyponatremia has been reported for decades [22, 27], but also with other first-generation antipsychotics such as chlorpromazine, perphenazine, and fluphenazine [23–25]. In the majority of cases there were other intercurrent factors involved in the development of hyponatremia (concomitant treatment with ACE inhibitors, diuretics and other psychotropic drugs).

3.2. Second generation antipsychotics (SGAS)

3.2.1. *Aripiprazole*

Aripiprazole is a partial agonist of dopamine, frequently used for its efficacy in cognitive and affective symptoms in psychosis. There are currently presentations for oral, parenteral and prolonged release treatment. Literature collects cases of aripiprazole-induced hyponatremia both in patients who developed the symptoms at the start of treatment [15] and in increasing the dose [26], improving in all of them the clinical symptoms with interruption of treatment and water restriction.

3.2.2. *Olanzapine*

It is an atypical antipsychotic, antagonist of D2 and 5HT2A receptor. It is commonly used in clinical practice to control agitation and positive symptoms. Cases of olanzapine-induced hyponatremia have been reported together with the concomitant use of other psychoactive drugs [5, 27]. In 2014, a case of death was described in a young schizophrenic male who presented with hyponatremia secondary to excessive water intake and which was related to the increase in the dose of olanzapine, which could have acted aggravating the intoxication itself [28].

3.2.3. *Quetiapine*

Synthesized in 1985, it is used in the treatment of schizophrenia, bipolar disorder, Alzheimer's disorder and major depression. There are few cases of SIADH induced by quetiapine, something that could be related to underdiagnosis and underreporting of this situation. Nonetheless, some cases are collected where quetiapine, together with other factors such as advanced age and polytherapy, is involved in the development of hyponatremia [29–31].

3.2.4. *Risperidone*

Approved by the FDA in 1993 for the use of schizophrenia, exists in oral presentation and depot. Like the other antipsychotics, risperidone has also been associated with the risk of developing hyponatremia, although some cases have been described in which the use of risperidone improved polydipsia in the schizophrenic patient [32, 33]. However, the results in the literature are inconclusive and controversial regarding the improvement of certain atypical antipsychotics (olanzapine and risperidone) on primary polidipsia.

3.2.5. *Paliperidone*

Paliperidone is an active metabolite of risperidone, indicated in the management of schizophrenia and schizoaffective disorder. In 2016, a case of rhabdomyolysis, malignant neuroleptic syndrome and SIADH associated with paliperidone prolonged release in a 35-year-old man hospitalized for psychotic decompensation was described. Two days after the administration of the treatment, the patient presented with a tonic-clonic seizure that was attributed to hypoosmolar hyponatremia [34]. It is important to remember that in all patients receiving antipsychotic treatment, serum sodium should be measured in the presence of epileptic seizures.

3.2.6. *Ziprasidone*

Ziprasidone is an atypical antipsychotic indicated in psychotic agitation, schizophrenia and manic and mixed episodes in bipolar disorder. The literature includes a series of cases in which hyponatremia is observed in the context of the use of ziprasidone, concomitantly with other psychopharmaceuticals such as duloxetine [35] and with comitial symptoms in the debut of the hyponatremia [36], as a neurological symptom present in cases of hyponatremia.

3.2.7. *Clozapine*

Synthesized in the late 1950s, clozapine is considered the first atypical antipsychotic. It emphasizes its low rate of extrapyramidal effects and its antipsychotic potency, being currently indicated in the management of resistant psychosis and psychotic symptoms in Parkinson's disease. Literature collects controversial data on its relationship with hyponatremia, although some authors defend its use in Syndrome of Psychosis, Intermittent Hyponatremia and Polydipsia (PIP syndrome) [37].

3.3. Syndrome of psychosis, intermittent hyponatremia and polydipsia (PIP syndrome)

Hyponatremia in psychotic patients is a relatively frequent complication, both due to the osmotic dysregulation of the disease and the secondary effect of antipsychotics. The PIP syndrome is characterized clinically by the presence of acute confusional symptoms derived from symptomatic hyponatremia and water intoxication. Between 6 and 20% of psychotic patients presents with polydipsia. In psychotic patients, in addition to xerostomia and consequent compulsive water intake, the role of supra-optic and paraventricular hypothalamic nuclei, responsible for the regulation of thirst and secretion of antidiuretic hormone (ADH) in the pathophysiology of hyponatremia, is postulated, as well as dopamine and endogenous opioids as neurotransmitters involved in the ingestion of water. Neuroimaging studies in schizophrenic patients show a ventricular dilation in basal conditions, however under conditions of hyponatremia cerebral edema and ventricular contraction are observed. Some studies show that the MDR1 C3435T polymorphism may increase the susceptibility to polydipsia in schizophrenia [38].

Despite its prevalence, morbidity and mortality, it is an underestimated entity in its prevention and early diagnosis. One of the diagnostic challenges is the differentiation between hyponatremia induced by antipsychotics and PIP, since often the treatment of one of the entities worsens the other. Some studies show that urine concentration measurements are useful to differentiate both situations, detecting more frequently concentrated urine in pharmacological hyponatremia and dilute urine secondary to psychotic decompensation [39]. While some studies show that clozapine can generate polydipsia and hyponatremia, others show that it improves the symptoms of polydipsia, so clozapine is postulated as a therapeutic option [37], especially as an alternative to electroconvulsive therapy in cases of catatonia [40].

4. Antidepressants

The consumption of antidepressants has increased significantly in most Organization for Economic Co-operation and Development (OECD) countries since the year 2000. There is significant variation in consumption of antidepressants between countries. For example, in Germany, antidepressant use had risen 46% in just 4 years, in case of Spain and Portugal, it rose about 20% during the same period and Iceland led the pack in overall use with about one in 10 people taking a daily antidepressant [41]. The new generation of antidepressant drugs are widely used as the first line of treatment for major depressive disorders and are considered to be safer than tricyclic agents due to a profile of better tolerability and lower rate of side effects [42]. Several side effects are transient and may disappear after a few weeks following treatment initiation, but potentially serious adverse events may persist or ensue later.

Hyponatramia is the most common electrolyte disorder in ambulatory outpatients, especially in the elderly, and is one of the many well-known side effects of antidepressants [43]. Most of the evidence pointing toward an increased risk of hyponatremia with the use of antidepressant medications is based on multiple case reports and a few observational studies. It is important to remember that mild hyponatremia is associated with instability and falls, reduced cognitive function, osteoporosis and increased morbidity and mortality [44]. Most studies are small and observational and only few have had the power to examine whether specific antidepressants carry a higher or lower risk of hyponatremia.

Hyponatremia, usually, is not dose dependent and the patient recovers when treatment with antidepressant is interrupted. For this reason, early detection as well as the evaluation of concomitant risk factors in all patients starting antidepressant are important. Besides, it seems necessary to supervise sodium plasma levels periodically when patients are in treatment with antidepressants and to choose safe drugs between all possibilities [45].

The selective serotonin reuptake inhibitors (SSRIs) and venlafaxine appear to be the antidepressants most commonly associated with hyponatremia. Between the SSRIs, the incidence of hyponatremia varies based on the definition of hyponatremia used. On the one hand, studies which defined hyponatremia as serum sodium levels <135 mmol/l, the incidence ranged from 9 to 40%. On the other hand, the incidence decreased to 0.06–2.6% when hyponatremia was defined as serum sodium levels <130 mmol/l. The number of case reports and small observational studies with hyponatremia concerning SSRI is substantially higher than the number of case reports and observational studies with other antidepressants, but it is not clear whether this is due to a true difference in incidence of hyponatremia. A review concluded that current evidence suggests a relatively higher risk of hyponatremia with SSRIs and venlafaxine compared to tricyclic antidepressants (TCA) and mirtazapine, but for several antidepressants, data were insufficient to determine the risk of hyponatremia [46]. We found that there were no consistent difference in the incidence of hyponatremia among different SSRI members, but available data indicate that the incidence could be slightly higher for citalopram, fluoxetine and escitalopram, whereas incidence rates may be lower for sertraline and paroxetine [47–49].

Nevertheless, according to national and international pharmacovigilance committees, 1/3 of the reports of drug induced hyponatremia are severe, with the greatest frequency involving paroxetine, fluoxetine, fluvoxamine, citalopram, venlafaxine, escitalopram and sertraline [50].

The data looking at the risk of hyponatremia associated with the use of serotonin–norepinephrine reuptake inhibitors (SNRIs) are even more limited. Most studies have found incidence rates of hyponatremia comparable to the ones reported for SSRIs. Incidence figures for mirtazapine and tricyclic antidepressants (TCAs) appear to be lower [46, 51].

The mechanisms of antidepressants induced hyponatremia remain incompletely elucidated, but these agents can act by either increasing the release of antidiuretic hormone (ADH) or increasing the sensitivity to ADH resulting in a clinical picture similar to the syndrome of inappropriate secretion of ADH [12]. It must be clarified that the precise mechanism is not known but today it is known that antidepressants are thought to cause the syndrome of inappropriate antidiuretic hormone release (SIADH) by direct or indirect stimulation of vasopressin release from the posterior pituitary gland. SIADH can be produced by multiple causes (hyponatremia with plasma hyposmolality and increased urinary excretion of sodium, increase in urinary osmolality, hypotension, heart failure, nephropathy, liver disease…) and lead to retention of water and to hyponatremia [52]. The prevalence of SIADH in patients using antidepressants has been described in several case reports and a case series and is estimated to occur in five of every 1000 patients treated per year [44, 46, 53–54]. If we take into account the genetic factor, it is known that most antidepressants are metabolized by the hepatic enzyme cytochrome P450 2D6 (CYP2D6), which is highly polymorphic with >60 variant alleles (http://www.cypalleles.ki.se). In case of individuals carrying two functional CYP2D6 alleles (**1, *2*) have "normal" enzyme activity and are classified as extensive metabolizers. However, 5–10% of the population lack enzyme activity due to inheritance of two nonfunctional alleles (**3, *4, *5, *6*) and form the so-called poor metabolizers. *CYP2D6*4* is the most common variant allele in Caucasians (allele frequency of 20%) [55]. Poor metabolizers have higher plasma concentrations of antidepressants metabolized by CYP2D6 and are therefore more likely to suffer from adverse drug events [56]. It has been hypothesized that hyponatraemia or low serum sodium concentration may be one of these adverse events [57]. This review evaluated the literature on association of hyponatremia and the different families of antidepressants.

4.1. SSRI: selective serotonin reuptake inhibitors

The phenomenon of recurrent hyponatremia induced by the use of SSRI has been described in the literature by some authors in subjects who were exposed to it.

Sertraline: In 2013 there were over 41 million prescriptions, making it the most prescribed antidepressant and second most prescribed psychiatric medication in the United States [58] and is used for a number of conditions. There are many publications with patient cases that take this treatment and suffer from hyponatremia [59, 60].

Paroxetine: Paroxetine is primarily used for many mental disorders, has a well-known discontinuation syndrome and shares many of the common adverse effects of SSRIs such as hyponatremia [61–63].

Fluoxetine: It is a widely used antidepressant, with a multitude of indications and has been assessed as the most effective and safe medicine needed in a health system [64]. There are many cases of patients with hyponatremia taking this treatment [65].

Citalopram: This antidepressant has a good anxiolytic profile but some cases of hyponatremia were recorded [66, 67].

Escitalopram: Is the (*S*)-stereoisomer of the earlier medication citalopram, used in clinical practice and is related with cases of hyponatremia [68, 69].

Fluvoxamine: Antidepressant with some uses and some analgesic properties. Many cases of hyponatremia were related [70, 71].

4.2. SNRI: serotonin-norepinephrine reuptake inhibitors

Data looking at the risk of hyponatremia associated with the use of SNRIs are even more limited but some cases were described.

Venlafaxine: Drug widely used in daily clinical practice, with indications for mental disorders and painful pathology. Cases of hyponatremia were registered [72–74].

Duloxetine: Recommended as a first line agent for the treatment of chemotherapy-induced neuropathy and for fibromyalgia in the presence of mood disorders, in addition to other disorders. There are patient cases that take this treatment and suffer from hyponatremia [75, 76].

Desvenlafaxine: Desvenlafaxine is a synthetic form of the major active metabolite of venlafaxine and some cases of hyponatremia were registered [77].

4.3. Mirtazapine

It has noradrenergical and specific serotonergical antidepressant effect and it is more likely to cause weight gain and sleepiness than other treatments. Some cases of hyponatremia were described [14, 53–55], however, this antidepressant has not been associated with hyponatremia in all cases or with less power of association to this side effect [46, 49, 53, 60, 76, 78].

4.4. Bupropion

Is a norepinephrine-dopamine reuptake inhibitor (NDRI) primarily used as an antidepressant and smoking cessation aid and related with cases of hyponatremia [79, 80], but less than other antidepressants and that does not happen in all cases [51, 61].

4.5. Tricyclic antidepressants

Discovered in the early 1950s, they have number of uses, many of their side effects may be related to the antimuscarinic properties and cases of hyponatremia were registered [81], but with fewer registered cases than with other antidepressants [47, 49, 82].

4.6. Vortioxetine

New antidepressant so-called serotonin modulator and stimulator and two cases of patients with hyponatremia were registered [83].

4.7. Trazodone

Is a serotonin antagonist and reuptake inhibitor that is widely used for the treatment of depression and insomnia. We found controversial results for relationship between trazodone and hyponatremia: case reports in patients on treatment [84], some cases were reported in overdose [85] or articles which describe less power of association to this side effect [51].

4.8. Agomelatine

Agomelatine is a potent agonist at melatonin receptors and an antagonist at serotonin-2C (5-HT2C) receptors. Given the limited references of hyponatremia associated with agomelatine, it has been postulated as a therapeutic alternative in those patients with risk or a history of hyponatremia that require antidepressant treatment [5].

4.9. Mianserine

Mianserin is a tetracyclic antidepressant with serotonergic (5HT2, 5HT1c), histaminergic and adrenergic ($\alpha1$,$\alpha2$) inhibitory activity. Some studies report that the association of hyponatremia and mianserin is low [86].

5. Antiepileptics

Epilepsy is a group of neurological disorders characterized by epileptic seizures. It is estimated that nearly 40 million people have epilepsy [86], with differences between countries and age groups. The median incidence of epilepsy is around 50.4/100,000/year: 45.0 for high-income countries and 81.7 for low- and middle-income countries [87]. Incidence is highest in old age (>60 years of age), with an estimated 60–135 new cases per 100,000 older adults each year [87]. Antiepileptics are, usually, initiated as monotherapy for the treatment of epilepsy [88].

However, these drugs are also often used in treatment of nonepileptic conditions such as pain and psychiatric disorders, for this reason it is very common in clinical practice that we find antiepileptics associated with other drugs [89].

As with antidepressants, many cases of hyponatremia are associated with the use of antiepileptic drugs and have been reported and published. However, there are great differences between them [90]. Besides all this, it is important to differentiate cases of antiepileptic that induce asymptomatic hyponatremia and can be easily corrected [91] from cases of severe or symptomatic hyponatremia. Last ones are associated with various types of neurological damage: seizures, altered mentality, brain stem herniation, death, etc., [92]. Because hyponatremia frequently goes undiagnosed and untreated with associated risks, next we will talk about the effect of different antiepileptics in this electrolyte abnormality.

5.1. Phenytoin

This drug was approved by the FDA in 1953. It works by blocking voltage-sensitive sodium channels. It is one of the most used and affordable antiepileptics, with several presentations. Some cases of hyponatremia related to the use of this drug have been described [93], but with less intensity than with other antiepileptic drugs [94].

5.2. Carbamazepine

Is used primarily in the treatment of epilepsy, neuropathic pain, schizophrenia along with other medications and as a second line agent in bipolar disorder. Carbamazepine is on the World Health Organization's List of Essential Medicines, the most effective and safe medicines needed in a health system World Health Organization [70]. It has sodium channel blocking effect. There are many publications with patient cases that take this treatment and suffer from hyponatremia, so it is one of the antiepileptics most frequently associated with this side effect [90, 93, 95–97].

5.3. Oxcarbazepine

Is a structural derivative of carbamazepine and acts by blocking voltage-sensitive sodium channels. Its use can reduce the occurrence of epileptic episodes, and in psychiatry, has been shown to improve mood (option for add-on therapy in the treatment of bipolar disorder) and reduce anxiety. There is approximately a 25–30% chance of cross-reactivity between carbamazepine and oxcarbazepine. Number of cases of hyponatremia have been recorded with this treatment and with greater strength of association [49, 84, 90, 92, 98, 99].

5.4. Eslicarbazepine acetate

The active component, eslicarbazepine, stabilizes the inactive state of voltage-gated sodium channels (same mechanism of action as oxcarbazepine). This new antiepileptic has potential uses for the treatment of trigeminal neuralgia and bipolar disorder. Cases of hyponatremia were recorded [91, 100, 101].

5.5. Topiramate

Its therapeutic activity and medical indications are very extensive, probably related to multireceptorial effects: voltage-gated sodium channels, GABA-A, AMPA/kainate, high-voltage-activated calcium channels and carbonic anhydrase isoenzymes. Some cases of hyponatremia are related [85], but with less frequency than with other antiepileptic drugs [102].

5.6. Lamotrigine

Is a sodium channel blocking drug (inhibits voltage-sensitive sodium channels), suppress the release of glutamate and aspartate (two dominant excitatory neurotransmitters) and blocks L-, N-, and P- type calcium channels, among other receptor effects. It is used in several neurological and psychiatric disorders and patients with hyponatremia has been notified [90, 103].

5.7. Valproate

Acts through blockade of voltage-gated sodium channels and increased brain levels of gamma-aminobutyric acid (GABA). It is used as primary option to treat epilepsy, bipolar disorder and to prevent migraine headaches, and is included in the World Health Organization's List of Essential Medicines, the most effective and safe medicines needed in a health system [64]. Many cases of hyponatremia with Valproate's treatment were identified [90, 93, 104–106].

5.8. Gabapentin

Is used primarily to treat seizures and neuropathic pain, and is commonly used to treat anxiety and other disorders. Gabapentin bind to the $\alpha 2\delta$-1 subunit of voltage-gated calcium channels, interacts with NMDA receptors, protein kinase C and inflammatory cytokines. There is little relationship between hyponatremia and the use of this drug [90].

5.9. Levetiracetam

This antiepileptic is used to treat epilepsy and different types of seizures. It also associates a multitude of indications for its use: Tourette syndrome, anxiety disorder, neuropathic pain… It acts as a neuromodulator binding to a synaptic vesicle glycoprotein (SV2A) and by inhibiting presynaptic calcium channels. Association of some cases of hyponatremia and use of levetiracetam has been documented [90, 107].

5.10. Pregabalin

It is useful when added to other treatments for many indications. It is an analog of GABA and increases the density of GABA transporter proteins, the rate of functional GABA transport and the extracellular GABA concentrations. Few cases of hyponatremia with use of pregabalin were reported [108].

6. Conclusions

Hyponatremia is a frequent clinical situation in clinical practice, both in outpatient and inpatient settings. Clinical manifestations have a broad spectrum with effect on different indicators such as morbidity and mortality. Nevertheless, this side effect is avoidable and reversible. Given the wide use of psychotropic drugs (antidepressants, antipsychotics and antiepileptics) and its current growing use, it is important to know those pharmacological options with lower risk of hyponatremia such as bupropion, trazodone, mianserin, pregabalin or gabapentin.

We have seen that etiology of hyponatremia is multifactorial and involves pharmacological origin (increase in the production or potentiation of the effects of antidiuretic hormone, alteration of the homeostasis of sodium and water), but many other factors such as advanced age, associated pathologies, female sex, weight or use of concomitant drugs also contribute to the development of hyponatremia. It is important to identify vulnerable patients and to measure sodium levels frequently, especially in the first few days after initiating treatment to help prevent or correct hyponatremia and its undesirable effects.

Conflict of interest

The authors declare no conflict of interests.

Author details

Mireia Martínez Cortés* and Pedro Gurillo Muñoz

*Address all correspondence to: mireia.martinez.cortes@gmail.com

Service of Psychiatry, Hospital Marina Baixa, Alicante, Spain

References

[1] Liamis G, Mitrogianni Z, Liberopoulos E, Tsimihodimos V, Elisaf M. Electrolyte disturbances in patients with hyponatremia. Internal Medicine. 2007;**46**(11):685-690

[2] Hoorn EJ, Lindemans J, Zietse R. Development of hypontraemia in hospitalized patients: Treatment-related risk factors and inadequate management. Nephrology, Dialysis, Transplantation. 2006;**21**(1):70-76

[3] Pham PC, Pham PM, Pham PT. Vasopressin excess and hyponatremia. American Journal of Kidney Diseases. 2006;**47**(5):727-737

[4] Waikar SS, Mount DB, Curhan GC. Mortality after hospitalization with mild, moderate and severe hiponatremia. The American Journal of Medicine. 2009 Sep;**122**(9):857-865

[5] Martínez Cortes M, Ogando Portilla N, Pecino Esquerdo B, Pérez MV. Antidepressant induced recurrent hyponatremia: A case report. Actas Españolas de Psiquiatría. 2013; **41**(6):361-364

[6] Gómez-Restrepo C, Bohórquez A, Pinto Masis D, Gil Laverde JFA, Rondon Sepúlveda M, Díaz-Granados N. Prevalencia de depresión y factores asociados con ella en la población. Pan American Journal of Public Health. 2004;**16**(6)

[7] Spasovski G et al. Clinical practice guideline on diagnosis and treatment of hyponatraemia. Nephrology, Dialysis, Transplantation. 2014;**29**(Suppl. 2):ii1-ii39. DOI: 10.1093/ndt/gfu040

[8] Rodríguez Padrón D, Carreta Iset MI, Pérez Leyva E, López Pereira L, Hernández García A, Velazco Silva E. Influencia de las acuaporinas en la génesis de múltiples enfermedades. Correo Cientifico Médico. Holguín abr-jun 2014;**18**(2)

[9] Corral Corral C, Quereda Rodríguez-Navarro C. Hiponatremia y sistema nervioso. Nefrologia Suplemento Extraordinario. 2011;**2**:48-60. DOI: 10.3265/Nefrologia Suplemento Extraordinario.pre2011.Sep.11148

[10] DeVita MV, Gardenswartz MH, Konecky A, Zabetakis PM. Incidence and etiology of hyponatremia in an intensive care unit. Clinical Nephrology. 1990;**34**(4):163-166

[11] Grikiniene J, Volbekas V, Stakisaitis D. Gender differences of sodium metabolism and hiponatremia as an adverse drug effect. Medicina (Kaunas, Lithuania). 2004;**40**(10):935-942

[12] Correll CU, Detraux J, De Lepeleire J, De Hert M. Effects of antipsychotics, antidepressants and mood stabilizers on risk for physical diseases in people with schizophrenia, depression and bipolar disorder. World Psychiatry. 2015;**14**:119-136. DOI: 10.1002/wps.20204

[13] Adrogue HJ, Madias NE. The Challengte of hyponatremia. Journal of the American Society of Nephrology. 2012;**23**:1140-1148. DOI: 10.1681/ASN.2012020128

[14] Montastruc F, Bénard-Laribière A, Noize P, et al. Antipsychotics use: 2006-2013 trends in prevalence and incidence and characterization of users. European Journal of Clinical Pharmacology. 06 Jan 2018;**74**(5):619-626. DOI: 10.1007/s00228-017-2406-0

[15] Kohen I, Voelker S, Manu P. Antipsychotic–induced hyponatremia: Case report and literature review. American Journal of Therapeutics. 2008;**15**:492. DOI: 10.1097/MJT.0b013e31817276e9

[16] Meulendijks D, Mannesse CK, Jansen PAF, van Marum RJ, Egberts TCG. Antipsychotic-induced hyponatraemia. A systematic review of the published evidence. Drug Safety. 2010;**33**:101-111

[17] Mannesse CK, van Puijenbroek EP, Jansen PA, van Marum RJ, Souverein PC, Egberts TC. Hyponatremia as an adverse drug reaction of antipsychotic drugs: A case-control study in VigBase. Drug Safety Jul 1, 2010;**33**(7):569-578. DOI: 10.2165/11532560-000000000-00000

[18] Manu P, Ray K, Rein JL, De Hert M, Kane JM, Correll CU. Medical outcome of psychiatric inpatients with admission hiponatremia. Türk Psikiyatri Dergisi. Summer 2011; **22**(2):123-125

[19] Yang HJ, Cheng WJ. Antipsychotic use is a risk factor for hyponatremia in patients with schizophrenia: A 15-year follow-up study. Psychopharmacology. Mar 2017;**234**(5):869-876. DOI: 10.1007/s00213-017-4525-9 Epub Jan 11, 2017

[20] Gandhi S, McArthur E, Reiss JP, Mamdanj MM, Hackam DG, Weir MA, Garg AX. Atypical antipsychotic medications and hyponatremia in older adults: A population-based cohort study. Canadian Journal of Kidney Health and Disease. Apr 11, 2016;**3**:21. DOI: 10.1186/s40697-016-0111-z (eCollection 2016)

[21] Josiassen RC, Curtis J, Filmyer DM, Audino B, Skuban N, Shaughnessy RA. Tolvaptan: A new tool for the effective treatment of hyponatremia in psychotic disorders. Expert Opinion on Pharmacotherapy. Mar 2010;**11**(4):637-648. DOI: 10.1517/14656561003610656

[22] Peck V, Shenkman L. Haloperidol-induced síndrome of inappropriate secretion of antidiuretic hormone. Clinical Pharmacology and Therapeutics. Oct 1979;**26**(4):442-444

[23] Ramasamy I. Severe hyponatraemia during therapy with ramipril. BMJ Case Reports. 2009. DOI: 10.1136/bcr.06.2009.1932

[24] Spigset O, Hedenmalm K. Hyponatremia during treatment with clomipramine, perphenazine, or clozapine: Study of therapeutic drug monitoring samples. Journal of Clinical Psychopharmacology. Oct 1996;**16**(5):412-414

[25] Vucicevic Z, Degoricija V, Alfirevic Z, Vukicevic-Badouin D. Fatal hiponatremia and other metabolic disturbances associated with pychotropic drug polypharmacy. International Journal of Clinical Pharmacology and Therapeutics. May 2007;**45**(5):289-292

[26] Yam FK, Jackson EA, Kwan BK. Syndrome of inappropriate antidiuretic hormone associated with aripiprazole. American Journal of Health-System Pharmacy. Dec 1, 2013; **70**(23):2110-2114. DOI: 10.2146/ajhp130142

[27] Bakhla AK, Guria RT, Kumar A. A suspected case of olanzapina induced hiponatremia. Indian Journal of Pharmacology. Jul–Aug 2014;**46**(4):441-442. DOI: 10.4103/0253-7613.135961

[28] Nagasawa S, Yajima D, Torimitsu S, Abe H, Iwase H. Fatal water intoxication during olanzapine treatment: A case report. Journal of Child and Adolescent Psychopharmacology. Dec 2013;**23**(10):699-700. DOI: 10.1089/cap.2013.0055

[29] Atalay A, Turhan N, Aki OE. A challenging case of syndrome of inappropriate secretion of antidiuretic hormone in an elderly patient secondary to quetiapine. Southern Medical Journal. 2007;**100**(8):832-833. DOI: 10.1097/SMJ.0b013e3180f607cf

[30] van den Heuvel OA, Bet PM, van Dam EW CM, Eeckhout AM. The syndrome of inappropriate antidiuretic hormone secretion (SIADH) during treatment with the antipsychotic agents haloperidol and quetiapine. Nederlands Tijdschrift voor Geneeskunde. 2006;**150**(35):1944-1948

[31] Theocharis K. Quetiapine-induced syndrome of inappropriate secretion of antidiuretic hormone. Case Reports in Psychiatry. 2016;**2016**:4803132. DOI: 10.1155/2016/4803132

[32] Rao N, Venkatasubramanian G, Korpade V, Behere R, Varambally S, Gangadhar B. Risperidone treatment for polidipsia and hiponatremia in schizophrenia: A case report. Türk Psikiyatri Dergisi. Summer 2011;**22**(2):123-125

[33] Whitten JR, Ruehter VL. Risperidone and hypontramia: A case report. Annals of Clinical Psychiatry. Sep 1997;**9**(3):181-183

[34] Kaur J, Kumar D, Alfishawy M, Lopez R, Sachmechi I. Paliperidone inducing concomitantly syndrome of inappropriate antidiuretic hormone. Case Reports in Critical Care. 2016;**2016**:2587963. DOI: 10.1155/2016/2587963

[35] Li RM, Wang C, Liu ZW, Zhao B. A case of severe hiponatremia induced by duloxetine and ziprasidone. Chinese Medical Journal. Oct 2012;**125**(20):3750-3751

[36] Akkaya C, An SA, Sivrioglu EY, Kotan Z, Kirli S. A patient using ziprasidone with polydipsia, seizure, hyponatremia and rhabdomyolisis. Progress in Neuro-Psychopharmacology & Biological Psychiatry. Dec 30, 2006;**30**(8):1535-1538. DOI: 10.1016/j.pnpbp.2006.05.020

[37] Diniz JB, Cordeiro Q, Zung S. Clozapine treatment for schizophrenia-related polydipsia. Revista Brasileira de Psiquiatria. Sep 2010;**32**(3):318-319

[38] Shinkai T, De Luca V, Utsunomiya K, Sakata S, Inoue Y, Fukunaka Y, Hwang R, Ohmori O, Kennedy JL, Nakamura J. Functional polymorphism of the human multidrug resistance gene (MDR1) and polydipsia-hyponatremia in schizophrenia. Neuromolecular Medicine. 2008;**10**(4):362-367. DOI: 10.1007/s12017-008-8041-2

[39] Atsariysing W, Goldman MB. A systematic review of the abilify of urine concentration to distinguish antipsychotic-from psychosis-induced hiponatremia. Psychiatry Research. Jul 30, 2014;**129**(3):217-233. DOI: 10.1016/j.psychres.2014.03.021

[40] Virk I, Dabo S, Ogunlesi CY, Olupona T, Akerele E. Treatment of catatonic schizophrenia and psychogenic polydipsia with clozapine: A case report. MOJ Addiction Medicine & Therapy. 2016;**2**(1):00015. DOI: 10.15406/mojamt.2016.02.00015

[41] OECD. Antidepressant drugs consumption, 2000 and 2015 [Internet]. 2017. Available from: http://www.oecd-ilibrary.org/social-issues-migration-health/health-at-a-glance-2017/antidepressant-drugs-consumption-2000-and-2015-or-nearest-year_health_glance-2017-graph181-en [Accessed: Feb 12, 2018]

[42] Agius M, Bonnici H. Antidepressants in use in clinical practice. Psychiatria Danubina. 2017;**29**(3):667-671

[43] Gartlehner G, Thieda P, Hansen RA, et al. Comparative risk for harms of second-generation antidepressants: A systematic review and meta-analysis. Drug Safety. 2008;**31**:851-865. DOI: 10.2165/00002018-200831100-00004

[44] Gunathilake R, Oldmeadow C, McEvoy M, et al. Mild hyponatremia is associated with impaired cognition and falls in community-dwelling older persons. Journal of the American Geriatrics Society. 2013;**61**:1838-1839. DOI: 10.1111/jgs.12468

[45] Región de Murcia. Boletín de Farmacovigilancia, 22. Hiponatremia por medicamentos [Internet]. 2011. Available from: http://www.murciasalud.es/recursos/ficheros/233703-boletin_22.pdf [Accesed: Feb 22, 2018]

[46] de Picker L, van, Den Eede F, Dumont G, et al. Antidepressants and the risk of hyponatremia: A class-byclass review of literature. Psychosomatics. 2014;**55**:536-547

[47] Coupland C, Dhiman P, Morriss R, et al. Antidepressant use and risk of adverse outcomes in older people: Population based cohort study. British Medical Journal. 2011;**343**:d4551. DOI: 10.1136/bmj.d4551

[48] Degner D, Grohmann R, Kropp S, et al. Severe adverse drug reactions of antidepressants: Results of the German multicenter drug surveillance program AMSP. Pharmacopsychiatry. 2004;**37**(1):S39-S45

[49] Letmaier M, Painold A, Holl AK, et al. Hyponatraemia during psychopharmacological treatment: Results of a drug surveillance programme. The International Journal of Neuropsychopharmacology. 2012;**15**(6):739-748. DOI: 10.1017/S1461145711001192

[50] Medicines Safety Update. Drug-Induced Hyponatraemia [Internet]. 2011. Available from: https://www.tga.gov.au/publication-issue/medicines-safety-update-vol-2-no-2-april-2011 [Accessed: Feb 27, 2018]

[51] Viramontes TS, Truong H, Linnebur SA. Antidepressant-induced hyponatremia in older adults. The Consultant Pharmacist®. 2016;**31**(3):139-150. DOI: 10.4140/TCP.n.2016.139

[52] Chan TY. Drug-induced syndrome of inappropriate antidiuretic hormone secretion. Causes, diagnosis and management. Drugs & Aging. 1997;**11**(1):27-24

[53] Farmand S, Lindh JD, Calissendorff J, et al. Differences in associations of antidepressants and hospitalization due to hyponatremia. The American Journal of Medicine. 2018;**131**(1):56-63. DOI: 10.1016/j.amjmed.2017.07.025

[54] Twardowschy CA, Bertolucci CB, Gracia CM, et al. Severe hyponatremia and the syndrome of inappropriate secretion of antidiuretic hormone (SIADH) associated with fluoxetine: Case report. Arquivos de Neuro-Psiquiatria. 2006;**64**:142-145. DOI: 10.1590/S0004-282X2006000100031

[55] Bradford LD. CYP2D6 allele frequency in European Caucasians, Asians, Africans and their descendants. Pharmacogenomics. 2002;**3**:229-243. DOI: 10.1517/14622416.3.2.229

[56] Bijl MJ, Visser LE, Hofman A, et al. Influence of the CYP2D6*4 polymorphism on dose, switching and discontinuation of antidepressants. British Journal of Clinical Pharmacology. 2008;**65**:558-564. DOI: 10.1111/j.1365-2125.2007.03052.x

[57] Kwadijk-de Gijsel S, Bijl MJ, Visser LE, et al. Variation in the CYP2D6 gene is associated with a lower serum sodium concentration in patients on antidepressants. British Journal of Clinical Pharmacology. 2009;**68**(2):221-225. DOI: 10.1111/j.1365-2125.2009.03448.x

[58] Grohol J. Top 25 Psychiatric Medication Prescriptions for 2013. Psych Central. Retrieved on June 16, 2018, from https://psychcentral.com/lib/top-25-psychiatric-medication-prescriptions-for-2013

[59] Raphael K, Tokeshi J. Hyponatremia associated with sertraline and fluoxetine: A case report. Hawaii Medical Journal. 2002;**61**(3):46-47

[60] Seshadri M, Thalitaya MD, Simon T, et al. Antidepressants and hyponatremia in a patient with colectomy–a case report. Psychiatria Danubina. 2017;**29**(3):610-614

[61] Piñón MV, Adán-Manes J. Selective serotonin reuptake inhibitor-induced hyponatremia: Clinical implications and therapeutic alternatives. Clinical Neuropharmacology. 2017;**40**(4):177-179

[62] Suwa A, Wakeno M, Tajika A, et al. Syndrome of inappropriate secretion of anti-diuretic hormone in an elderly depressive patient receiving paroxetine: A case report. International Journal of Geriatric Psychiatry. 2010;**25**(4):433-434

[63] Koide T, Wakabayashi T, Matsuda T, et al. Hyponatremia associated with paroxetine induced by sodium-restricted diet and hypotonic saline. Pharmacy World & Science. 2010;**32**(1):19. DOI: 10.1007/s11096-009-9353-5

[64] World Health Organization. WHO Model List of Essential Medicines, 20th List [Internet]. 2017. Available from: http://www.who.int/entity/medicines/publications/essential-medicines/20th_EML2017_FINAL_amendedAug2017.pdf?ua=1 [Accessed: Mar 1, 2018]

[65] Kaya T, Yücel M, Eraslan Ö, et al. Severe hyponatremia, epistaxis, and fluoxetine. Journal of Ayub Medical College Abbottabad. 2016;**28**(1):204-205

[66] Leth-Møller KB, Hansen AH, Torstensson M, et al. Antidepressants and the risk of hyponatremia: A Danish register-based population study. BMJ Open. 2016;**6**(5):e011200

[67] Richter T, Paluch Z, Alusik S. The non-antidepressant effects of citalopram: A clinician's perspective. Neuroendocrinology Letters. 2014;**35**(1):7-12

[68] Rawal G, Kumar R, Yadav S. Severe hyponatremia associated with escitalopram. Journal of Family Medicine and Primary Care. 2017;**6**(2):453. DOI: 10.4103/2249-4863.220043

[69] Vidyasagar S, Rao K, Verma M, et al. Escitalopram induced SIADH in an elderly female: A case study. Psychopharmacology Bulletin. 2017;**47**(4):52

[70] Gabriel A. Serotonin reuptake inhibitor and fluvoxamine-induced severe hyponatremia in a 49-year-old man. Case Reports in Medicine. 13 Oct 2009;**2009**:585193. (PMID:19829765 PMCID:PMC2761047). DOI: 10.1155/2009/585193

[71] Inaguma D, Kitagawa W, Hayashi H, et al. Three cases of severe hyponatremia under taking selective serotonin reuptake inhibitor (SSRI). Nihon Jinzo Gakkai Shi. 2000;**42**(8): 644-648

[72] Delucia B. Naltrexone for self-injury in borderline personality with venlafaxine-associated hyponatremia. Journal of Clinical Psychopharmacology. 2017;**37**(6):743-745. DOI: 10.1097/JCP.0000000000000781

[73] Grover S, Somaiya M, Ghormode D. Venlafaxine-associated hyponatremia presenting with catatonia. The Journal of Neuropsychiatry and Clinical Neurosciences. 2013; **25**(2):E11-E12. DOI: 10.1176/appi.neuropsych.12030070

[74] Revol R, Rault C, Polard E, et al. Hyponatremia associated with SSRI/NRSI: Descriptive and comparative epidemiological study of the incidence rates of the notified cases from the data of the French National Pharmacovigilance Database and the French National Health Insurance. L'Encephale. June 2018;**44**(3):291-296. DOI: 10.1016/j.encep.2017.09.003. [Epub 2017 Dec 14]

[75] Kulkarni M. Duloxetine induced hyponatremia. Indian Journal of Nephrology. 2015; **25**(4):259. DOI: 10.4103/0971-4065.151352

[76] Liew ED, Alderman CP. Syndrome of inappropriate antidiuretic hormone secretion associated with desvenlafaxine. International Journal of Clinical Pharmacy. 2014;**36**(2):253-255. DOI: 10.1007/s11096-013-9870-0

[77] Fernández EG, García DR. Syndrome of inappropriate antidiuretic hormone secretion associated with desvenlafaxine. European Psychiatry. 2016;**33**:S581

[78] Ghosh A, Hegde A, Grover S. Mirtazapine-associated hyponatremia presenting as delirium. Indian Journal of Pharmacology. 2014;**46**(4):448

[79] Kate N, Grover S, Kumar S, et al. Bupropion-induced hyponatremia. General Hospital Psychiatry. 2013;**35**(6):681-e11. DOI: 10.1016/j.genhosppsych.2013.04.020

[80] Kim CS, Choi JS, Bae EH, et al. Hyponatremia associated with bupropion. Electrolytes & Blood Pressure. 2011;**9**(1):23-26. DOI: 10.5049/EBP.2011.9.1.23

[81] Paksu S, Duran L, Altuntas M, et al. Amitriptyline overdose in emergency department of university hospital: Evaluation of 250 patients. Human & Experimental Toxicology. 2014;**33**(9):980-990. DOI: 10.1177/0960327113520019

[82] Sultana J, Spina E, Trifirò G. Antidepressant use in the elderly: The role of pharmacodynamics and pharmacokinetics in drug safety. Expert Opinion on Drug Metabolism & Toxicology. 2015;**11**(6):883-892. DOI: 10.1517/17425255.2015.1021684

[83] Pelayo-Terán JM, Martínez-Pérez MM, Zapico-Merayo Y. Safety in the use of antidepressants: Vortioxetine-induce hyponatremia in a case report. Revista de Psiquiatria y Salud Mental. 2017;**10**(4):219-220

[84] Lange-Asschenfeldt C, Kojda G, Cordes J, et al. Epidemiology, symptoms, and treatment characteristics of hyponatremic psychiatric inpatients. Journal of Clinical Psychopharmacology. 2013;**33**(6):799-805

[85] Avila JD. Fatal cerebral edema, seizures, and hyponatremia after trazodone overdose. Clinical Neuropharmacology. 2017;**40**(5):221-223. DOI: 10.1097/WNF.0000000000000235

[86] Vos T, Allen C, Arora M, et al. Global, regional, and national incidence, prevalence, and years lived with disability for 310 diseases and injuries, 1990-2015: A systematic analysis for the global burden of disease study 2015. The Lancet. 2016;**388**(10053):1545-1602

[87] Leppik IE. Treatment of epilepsy in the elderly. Current Treatment Options in Neurology. 2008;**10**:239-245. DOI: 10.1046/j.1535-7597.2001.00013.x

[88] Glauser T, Ben-Menachem E, Bourgeois B, et al. ILAE treatment guidelines: Evidence-based analysis of antiepileptic drug efficacy and effectiveness as initial monotherapy for epileptic seizures and syndromes. Epilepsia. 2006;**47**:1094-1120. DOI: 10.1111/j.1528-1167.2006.00585.x

[89] Geller AI, Nopkhun W, Dows-Martinez MN, et al. Polypharmacy and the role of physical medicine and rehabilitation. PMR. March 2012;**4**(3):198-219. DOI: 10.1016/j.pmrj.2012.02.012

[90] Lu X, Wang X. Hyponatremia induced by antiepileptic drugs in patients with epilepsy. Expert Opinion on Drug Safety. 2017;**16**(1):77-87. DOI: 10.1080/14740338.2017.1248399

[91] Gupta DK, Bhoi SK, Kalita J, et al. Hyponatremia following esclicarbazepine therapy. Seizure-European Journal of Epilepsy. 2015;**29**:11-14. DOI: 10.1016/j.seizure.2015.03.005

[92] Kim YS, Kim DW, Jung KH, et al. Frequency of and risk factors for oxcarbazepine-induced severe and symptomatic hyponatremia. Seizure-European Journal of Epilepsy. 2014;**23**(3):208-212. DOI: 10.1016/j.seizure.2013.11.015

[93] Gandhi S, McArthur E, Mamdani MM, et al. Antiepileptic drugs and hyponatremia in older adults: Two population-based cohort studies. Epilepsia. 2016;**57**(12):2067-2079. DOI: 10.1111/epi.13593

[94] Okamoto M, Nako Y, Tachibana A, et al. Efficacy of phenytoin against hyponatremic seizures due to SIADH after administration of anticancer drugs in a neonate. Journal of Perinatology. 2002;**22**(3):247. DOI: 10.1038/sj.jp.7210657

[95] Sekiya N, Awazu M. A case of nephrogenic syndrome of inappropriate antidiuresis caused by carbamazepine. CEN Case Reports. May 2017;**7**(1):66-68. DOI: 10.1007/s13730-017-0295-9. [Epub 2017 Dec 27]

[96] Berghuis B, Palen J, Haan GJ, et al. Carbamazepine-and oxcarbazepine-induced hyponatremia in people with epilepsy. Epilepsia. 2017;**58**(7):1227-1233

[97] Fuseya Y, Komatsu K, Matsumoto S. Transient Splenial lesion following abrupt withdrawal of carbamazepine. Internal Medicine. 2017;**56**(8):989-990. DOI: 10.2169/internalmedicine.56.7910

[98] Druschky K, Bleich S, Grohmann R, et al. Use and safety of antiepileptic drugs in psychiatric inpatients—Data from the AMSP study. European Archives of Psychiatry and Clinical Neuroscience. 2018;**268**(2):191-208

[99] Kellinghaus C, Berning S, Stögbauer F. Use of oxcarbazepine for treatment of refractory status epilepticus. Seizure-European Journal of Epilepsy. 2014;**23**(2):151-154. DOI: 10.1016/j.seizure.2013.11.002

[100] Gama H, Vieira M, Costa R, et al. Safety profile of eslicarbazepine acetate as add-on therapy in adults with refractory focal-onset seizures: From clinical studies to 6 years of post-marketing experience. Drug Safety. 2017;**40**(12):1231-1240. DOI: 10.1007/s40264-017-0576-4

[101] Toledano R, Jovel CE, Jiménez-Huete A, et al. Efficacy and safety of eslicarbazepine acetate monotherapy for partial-onset seizures: Experience from a multicenter, observational study. Epilepsy & Behavior. 2017;**73**:173-179. DOI: 10.1016/j.yebeh.2017.02.028

[102] Sommer BR, Fenn HH, Ketter TA. Safety and efficacy of anticonvulsants in elderly patients with psychiatric disorders: Oxcarbazepine, topiramate and gabapentin. Expert Opinion on Drug Safety. 2007;**6**(2):133-145. DOI: 10.1517/14740338.6.2.133

[103] Mewasingh L, Aylett S, Kirkham F, et al. Hyponatraemia associated with lamotrigine in cranial diabetes insipidus. The Lancet. 2000;**356**(9230):656. DOI: 10.1016/S0140-6736(00)02613-1

[104] Wu XT, Hong PW, Suolang DJ, et al. Drug-induced hypersensitivity syndrome caused by valproic acid as a monotherapy for epilepsy: First case report in Asian population. Epilepsy & Behavior Case Reports. 2017;**8**:108-110. DOI: 10.1016/j.ebcr.2017.06.003

[105] Gupta E, Kunjal R, Cury JD. Severe hyponatremia due to valproic acid toxicity. Journal of Clinical Medicine Research. 2015;**7**(9):717

[106] Patel KR, Meesala A, Stanilla JK. Sodium valproate–induced hyponatremia: A case report. Primary Care Companion to the Journal of Clinical Psychiatry. 2010;**12**(5):PCC.09l00941

[107] Rosca EC, Simu M. Levetiracetam-induced hyponatremia. Acta Neurologica Belgica. 28 Jul 2017;**118**(1):123-124. DOI: 10.1007/s13760-017-0825-4

[108] Jung YJ, Lee DY, Kim HW, et al. A case report of syndrome of inappropriate antidiuretic hormone induced by Pregabalin. Electrolytes & Blood Pressure. 2016;**14**(2):31-34. DOI: 10.5049/EBP.2016.14.2.31

Chapter 3

Metabolic Alkalosis

Holly Mabillard and John A. Sayer

Additional information is available at the end of the chapter

http://dx.doi.org/10.5772/intechopen.78724

Abstract

Metabolic alkalosis is a disorder where the primary defect, an increase in plasma bicarbonate concentration, leads to an increase in systemic pH. Here we review the causes of metabolic alkalosis with an emphasis on the inherited causes, namely Gitelman syndrome and Bartter syndrome and syndromes which mimic them. We detail the importance of understanding the kidney pathophysiology and molecular genetics in order to distinguish these syndromes from acquired causes. In particular we discuss the tubular transport of salt in the thick ascending limb of the loop of Henle, the distal convoluted tubule and the collecting duct. The effects of salt wasting, namely an increase in the renin-angiotensin-aldosterone axis are discussed in order to explain the biochemical phenotypes and targeted treatment approaches to these conditions.

Keywords: salt-wasting, inherited tubulopathy, renin-angiotensin-aldosterone axis

1. Introduction

Metabolic alkalosis is a disorder where the primary defect, an increase in plasma bicarbonate concentration, leads to an increase in systemic pH. Various mechanisms underpin the pathophysiology of metabolic alkalosis, which is defined by an arterial bicarbonate concentration of over 28 mmol/L or a venous total carbon dioxide concentration of greater than 30 mmol/L. The body compensates for alkali retention and subsequent elevated arterial pH by inducing respiratory hypoventilation resulting in an accompanying rise in $PaCO_2$. Normally the kidney, which has a protective mechanism against the development of significant increases in bicarbonate, will excrete excess alkali to restore the body to its homeostatic pH, but certain factors can impair this ability resulting in a sustained alkalotic state. Here we will review the pathophysiological mechanisms and clinical settings in which metabolic alkalosis may occur [1–4] and give an overview of the causes of the inherited forms of metabolic alkalosis. The importance of defining a molecular genetic cause of metabolic alkalosis is reviewed alongside the common mimics of some of the inherited metabolic alkalosis syndromes.

2. Pathophysiology of metabolic alkalosis

The following mechanisms result in the elevation of serum bicarbonate; excessive loss of hydrogen ions by the kidney or via the GI tract, intracellular shift of hydrogen ions, retention of exogenous bicarbonate ions or volume contraction around a constant supply of extracellular bicarbonate (contraction alkalosis) [5].

As water dissociates in the body to hydrogen and hydroxyl ions, the hydroxyl ions combine with carbon dioxide, resulting in bicarbonate, as hydrogen ions are removed from extracellular fluid. Hydrogen ion removal in the kidney and GI tract is accompanied by loss of potassium and chloride so hypokalaemia and hypochloraemia often coexist with metabolic alkalosis.

Ability to excrete excess bicarbonate depends on the normal function of nephrons within the kidneys. The kidney therefore is implicated in the pathophysiology of most forms of metabolic alkalosis. The following scenarios result in a degree of impairment of this important mechanism: hypovolaemia, reduced glomerular filtration rate (GFR), reduced effective arterial volume, hypokalaemia, hypochloraemia or hyperaldosteronism.

2.1. Volume depletion

Both reduced extracellular volume and arterial pressure will reduce GFR and thus activate the renin-angiotensin-aldosterone and sympathetic nervous system. Decreased GFR reduces bicarbonate filtration by the kidney and angiotensin and sympathetic activation increases bicarbonate reabsorption and generation in addition to sodium reabsorption in the tubule. This is done in the following ways:

- Angiotensin-2 stimulates apical sodium-hydrogen exchange and basolateral sodium bicarbonate co-transport in the proximal tubule. This increases bicarbonate and sodium reabsorption.
- In the apical membrane of alpha-intercalated cells of the collecting duct angiotensin-2 and aldosterone increase H^+-ATPase pump activity resulting in increased urinary excretion of hydrogen ions. This results in increased intracellular bicarbonate generation which exits the cell in exchange for chloride via the basolateral membrane.
- Increases in aldosterone stimulate the apically located ENaC channel in the principal cells, which generates an electronegative potential in the tubular lumen. This enhances hydrogen and potassium ion excretion.

2.2. Sodium intake

A low sodium chloride diet will increase the bicarbonate reabsorption in the kidney enough to elevate serum pH although the reverse is not true with a high salt diet even though this will encourage the kidney to excrete sodium bicarbonate.

http://dx.doi.org/10.5772/intechopen.78724

2.3. Chloride depletion

Chloride depletion secondary to vomiting or nasogastric suction leads to a metabolic alkalosis. Chloride depletion metabolic alkalosis causes concomitant potassium depletion through renal loss of potassium. A less severe chloride depletion metabolic alkalosis is seen with the use of thiazide and loop diuretics.

2.4. Hypokalaemia

Hypokalaemia causes alkalosis by moving hydrogen ions into the intracellular space in exchange for extracellular movement of potassium and hypokalaemia maintains an alkalosis by increasing renal bicarbonate reabsorption. Hypokalaemia (and aldosterone) stimulates the distal Na^+-K^+-ATPase and H^+-ATPase pumps in the apical membrane of alpha-intercalated cells to reabsorb potassium and secrete hydrogen and subsequently maintain alkalosis. Hypokalaemia also causes extracellular movement of potassium in exchange for intracellular movement of sodium and hydrogen which generates extracellular bicarbonate although co-existent intracellular acidosis. This intracellular acidosis stimulates renal bicarbonate reabsorption, hydrogen secretion and ammonium synthesis and excretion.

2.5. Increased aldosterone

Hyperaldosteronism in addition to increased distal tubule sodium delivery results in sodium reabsorption and hydrogen and potassium ion secretion. Any hyper-reninaemic state which will result in an increase in aldosterone production will have the same effects.

2.6. Volume contraction and beta-intercalated cells

Distal tubule chloride delivery is essential for the beta-intercalated cell to secrete bicarbonate as this occurs by an apical anion exchange protein called Pendrin (**Figure 3**). As volume contraction reduces distal chloride delivery, bicarbonate secretion will reduce as will chloride reabsorption. Urine pH becomes acidic with little chloride, sodium and potassium, so beta-intercalated cells are blunted from excreting bicarbonate and correcting the metabolic alkalosis [1–4].

3. Causes of metabolic alkalosis

3.1. Diuretics

Loop diuretics (Furosemide, Bumetanide, Torsemide) inhibit the apical Na^+–K^+–$2Cl^-$ co-transporter in the thick ascending limb of the loop of Henle where 20–25% of sodium is typically reabsorbed. Metabolic alkalosis occurs in several ways [6, 7]:

- Increased distal sodium delivery results in stimulation of the aldosterone sensitive sodium channel (ENaC) which increases hydrogen/potassium ion excretion.
- Hypochloraemia will also contribute to the metabolic alkalosis.

The same principle also applies to other diuretics such as thiazides.

3.2. Post-hypercapnia

Patients who are chronic CO_2 retainers typically develop a compensatory metabolic alkalosis due to renal bicarbonate retention. Once the hypercapnia is reversed with ventilatory support, the renal bicarbonate retention takes longer to correct and these patients usually have a chronically elevated bicarbonate [8].

3.3. Non-reabsorbable anion delivery

Antibiotics particularly Beta-lactams act as non-reabsorbable anions in the renal tubule which therefore promotes potassium and hydrogen excretion which results in metabolic alkalosis [9].

3.4. Inherited salt wasting alkaloses

Bartter and Gitelman syndromes are both autosomal recessive inherited disorders which result in characteristic features due to a hereditary dysfunction in a tubular salt handling [10]. Both result in hypokalaemia, metabolic alkalosis, hyper-reninaemia and hyperaldosteronism with low blood pressure. The prevalence of Gitelman syndrome is about 1 in 40,000 compared with Bartter syndrome, which has a prevalence of 1 in 1,000,000. Bartter syndrome is more severe and may cause perinatal death due to salt wasting crises. The clinical phenotype that is seen with Gitelman syndrome mimics the chronic ingestion of a thiazide diuretic and that of Bartter syndrome mimics a chronic loop diuretic effect (**Table 1**). Bartter and Gitelman syndrome carriers (heterozygous for a mutation in causative gene) typically have lower blood pressure than that of the general population and may have mild biochemical phenotypes and some clinical symptoms.

Bartter syndrome results from a primary defect in sodium chloride reabsorption in the thick ascending limb of the loop of Henle (**Figure 1**). Salt (sodium) wasting results in volume depletion which activates juxtaglomerular secretion of renin and subsequent juxtaglomerular hyperplasia and hyperaldosteronism. Volume depletion and increased distal tubular sodium delivery result in tubular potassium and hydrogen secretion in the urine [11, 12]. Paracellular reabsorption of calcium and magnesium in the thick ascending limb of the loop of Henle is driven by sodium chloride reabsorption in this nephron segment. Reduced sodium absorption here results in hypercalciuria and hypomagnesaemia [13].

To date, there are five types of Bartter syndrome based on different genetic defects (**Figure 1**) with slightly variable phenotypic presentations [14].

Type 1: mutations *SLC12A1* which encodes the apically located Na-K-2Cl (NKCC2) result in a severe phenotype which can cause maternal polyhydramnios and prematurity. Subsequently, few survive infancy due to extreme salt wasting resulting in significant hypokalaemia, metabolic alkalosis, polyuria and hypercalciuria.

Type 2: mutations in *KCNJ1*, which encodes the apical potassium channel ROMK essential for potassium recirculation in the thick ascending limb of the loop of Henle results in salt-wasting alkalosis. Nephrocalcinosis is common which often results in later renal dysfunction and, in some cases, end stage renal failure [15].

http://dx.doi.org/10.5772/intechopen.78724

	Bartter syndrome	Gitelman syndrome
Site of defect	NKCC2, ROMK, CLC-KB, CLC-KA and CaSR in the thick ascending limb of the loop of Henle	Apical sodium chloride co-transporter (NCCT) at the distal convoluted tubule
Metabolic alkalosis	Present	Present
Hypokalaemia	Present	Present
Hypocalcaemia	Rare (seen in Type 5 Bartter syndrome)	Absent
Hypomagnesaemia	Occasionally present	Present
Urine chloride and sodium excretion	High	Normal/high
Urine potassium excretion	Normal/high	High
Urine calcium excretion	Normal/high	Low
Urinary concentrating ability	Impaired	Normal
Urine prostaglandin excretion	High	Normal
Hyper-reninaemic Hyperaldosteronism	Present	Present
Age at presentation	Antenatal/neonatal periods	Childhood/adolescence/adult
Polyhydramnios	Common	Absent
Failure to thrive	Typically present	Absent
Growth retardation	Typically present	Rarely present
Polyuria and polydipsia	Present	Absent
Sensorineural deafness	Present in Type 4 Bartter syndrome	Absent
Chondrocalcinosis	Absent	Occasionally present
Nephrocalcinosis	Present in Type 1 and Type 2 Bartter syndrome	Absent
Muscle weakness/tetany	Occasionally present	Present

Table 1. Differences between Bartter and Gitelman syndrome.

Type 3: mutations in *CLCNKB* result in loss of function of the basolateral chloride channel ClC-Kb which is historically described as the 'classical' form of Bartter syndrome. This form is less severe and may present later in childhood. Co-expression of ClC-Ka results in a less severe phenotype. Some patients with *CLCNKB* mutations have a Gitelman syndrome phenotype with hypocalciuria and thiazide non-responsiveness because ClC-Kb is also involved with chloride reabsorption along the distal convoluted tubule in addition to the thick ascending limb of the loop of Henle. Late renal impairment can feature in this form of Bartter syndrome mainly due to nephrocalcinosis and the adverse effects of NSAIDS (used as treatment for the condition) [16].

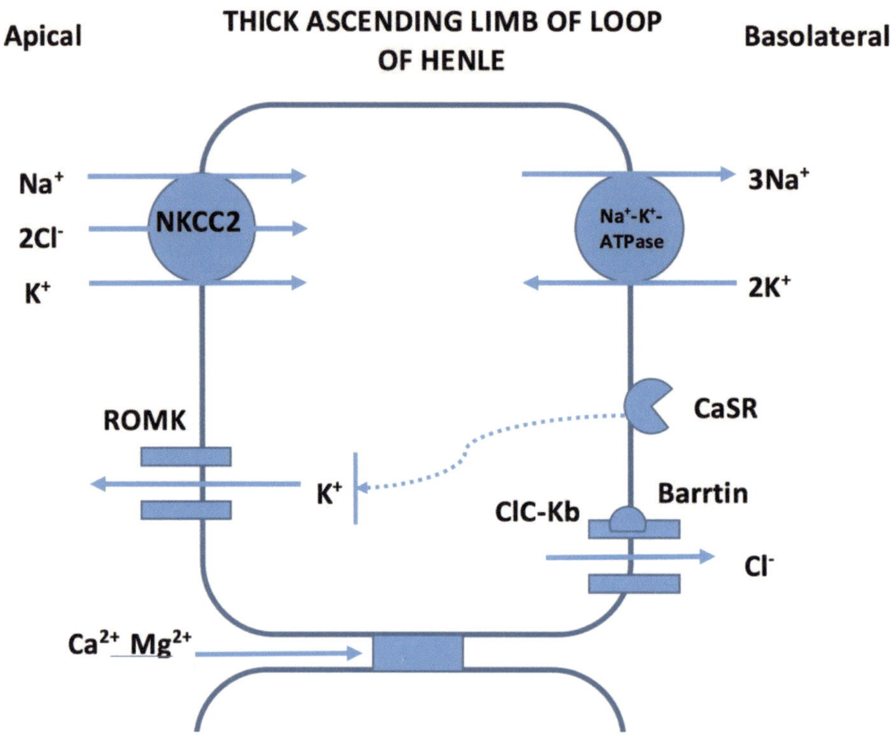

Figure 1. The thick ascending loop of Henle and the transporters and channels associated with tubulopathies.

Type 4: two mechanisms underlie type 4 Bartter syndrome. Both defects cause severe disease in the antenatal period and present with co-existent congenital deafness. Progressive renal failure is more common but nephrocalcinosis is less commonly seen. Type 4A is a consequence of a defect in the Barttin subunit that is essential to the function of both the chloride channels ClC-Ka and ClC-Kb which are present in both the renal tubule and the stria vascularis of the cochlear (inner ear). Bartter type 4b involves a second mechanism whereby digenic mutations affect both chloride channels (*CLCNKA* and *CLCNKB*) [17].

Type 5: this form of Bartter syndrome is due to a gain of function mutation in *CASR* encoding the calcium sensing receptor (CaSR). This is also termed autosomal dominant hypocalcaemia. This condition results in a low serum calcium as a result of downward 'resetting' of the parathyroid gland and hypocalcaemia subsequently inhibits parathyroid hormone release. The gain of function mutation in CaSR additionally regulates paracellular calcium transport in the thick ascending limb of the loop of Henle. CaSR over-activation reduces ROMK expression in addition to blunting Na^+–K^+–$2Cl^-$ co-transporter expression resulting in renal sodium chloride wasting. Calcium and magnesium reabsorption via paracellular channels is inhibited due to lack of electrochemical gradient to drive paracellular reabsorption. This Bartter syndrome subtype is unique due to the presence of hypocalcaemia and an autosomal dominant inheritance pattern and has a milder phenotype (with much less alkalosis) and with later onset [18].

A transient form of Bartter syndrome exists as an X-linked pattern of inheritance which manifests in the antenatal period. This form presents with severe polyhydramnios and prematurity

http://dx.doi.org/10.5772/intechopen.78724

if the foetus survives to this stage. Severe salt wasting results in foetal polyuria and those that survive to birth have spontaneous resolution in symptoms over the first few months/years of life. Mutations in *MAGED2*, which encodes melanoma-associated antigen D2, underlie this condition. The gene is thought to affect the antenatal expression and function of NKCC2 and NCC via adenylate cyclase, a cytoplasmic heat-shock protein and cyclic AMP [19].

The apically expressed furosemide sensitive co-transporter/sodium potassium chloride co-transporter (NKCC2) is shown. Mutations in Type 1 Bartter syndrome are associated with dysfunction in this channel, leading to salt wasting. Mutations in the apical potassium channel *ROMK* cause Type 2 Bartter syndrome. ROMK is essential for potassium recycling back to the lumen of the tubule in this nephron segment. Mutations in *CLCNKB* encoding the basolateral chloride channel ClC-Kb cause type 3 Bartter syndrome (as well as causing phenotypes similar to Gitelman syndrome). Type 4 Bartter syndrome is due to mutations in *BSND* which acts as a subunit for both ClC-Kb and ClC-Ka (not shown). *BSND* mutations also cause sensorineural deafness. The basolateral calcium-sensing receptor (CaSR) regulates ROMK and its overstimulation/gain of function causes an inhibition of ROMK, producing a Bartter-like phenotype. Calcium and magnesium are resorbed via paracellular channels, and any loss of the electrochemical driving force will lead to hypercalciuria and magnesium wasting. Dysfunction at this nephron segment leads to severe renal salt wasting, which activates the renin-angiotensin-aldosterone system. The increased delivery of salt to the cortical collecting duct promotes aldosterone dependant Na^+ reabsorption via ENaC, which is coupled to K^+ and H^+ secretion, thus accounting for the hypokalaemic alkalosis seen.

Gitelman syndrome differs from Bartter syndrome due to the presence of hypocalciuria and does not typically manifest until adolescence or adulthood. Differentiating Gitelman syndrome from Type 3 Bartter syndrome can be difficult [20] due to expression of CLCKNB in distal nephron segments as well as the thick ascending limb of the loop of Henle.

Gitelman syndrome results from inactivating mutations in *SLC12A3* which encodes the sodium chloride co-symporter (NCCT) (**Figure 2**) in the distal convoluted tubule [21]. The clinical phenotype can be variable and no phenotype-genotype correlation is yet understood. It is theorised that lack of correlation could be due to differences in function and/or expression of other basolateral chloride channels such as the voltage-gated chloride channel, KCl co-transporter or the cystic fibrosis transmembrane conductance regulator [22].

EAST syndrome (alias SeSAME, OMIM #612780) is causes by mutations in *KCNJ10*, a basolateral potassium channel (**Figure 2**) expressed in the distal convoluted tubule [23, 24]. Biochemically, the phenotype exactly mimics Gitelman syndrome. Extra-renal manifestations of epilepsy, ataxia and speech dyspraxia make the syndrome recognisable.

The apically expressed thiazide sensitive co-transporter/sodium chloride co-transporter (NCCT) is shown. Mutations in Gitelman syndrome are associated with dysfunction in this channel, leading to salt wasting. Mutations in the basolateral potassium channel *KCNJ10* cause EAST syndrome and the serum biochemistry phenotypically mimics Gitelman syndrome. This channel is required for potassium recycling from the Na^+–K^+–ATPAse. Mutations in *CLCNKB* encoding the basolateral chloride channel ClC-Kb can also mimic Gitelman syndrome (as well as causing Bartter syndrome). Dysfunction of the apical magnesium channel in the distal convoluted tubule encoded by *TRPM6* is seen in Gitelman syndrome, explaining

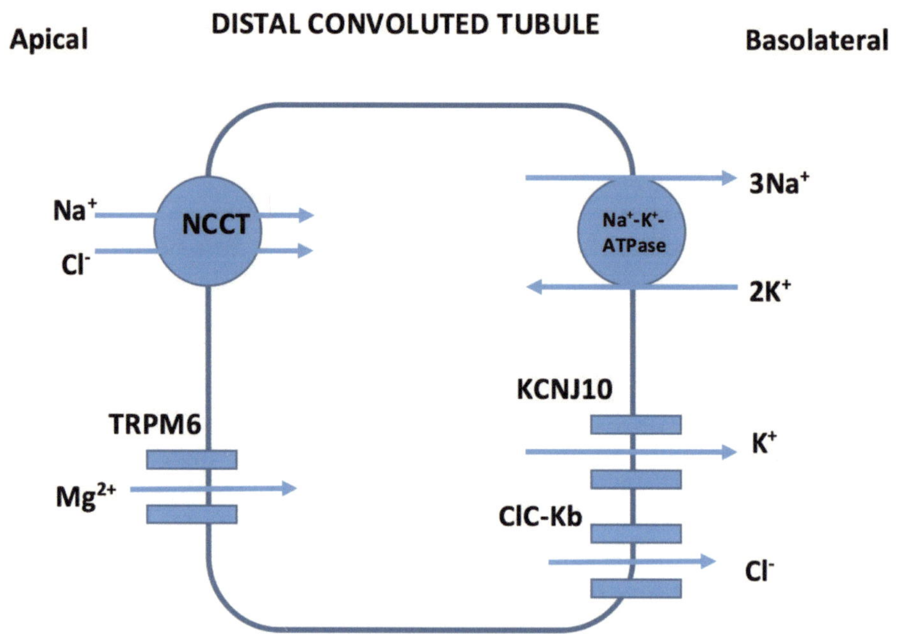

Figure 2. The distal convoluted tubule and the transporters and channels associated with tubulopathies.

the hypomagnesaemia. Renal salt loss activates the renin-angiotensin-aldosterone system and increased delivery of salt to the cortical collecting duct promotes aldosterone dependant Na^+ reabsorption via ENaC, which is coupled to K^+ and H^+ secretion, thus accounting for the hypokalaemic alkalosis seen.

Treatment for these in inherited salt wasting alkaloses conditions, in addition to electrolyte replacement, can comprise of NSAIDs, typically indomethacin. Renal production of PGE2 is typically elevated in response to reduced entry of chloride into the macula densa in the end of the thick ascending limb in these conditions [25]. Cyclooxygenase 2 expression is subsequently increased. PGE2 stimulates renin release by the juxtaglomerular apparatus contributing to the phenotype. PGE2 synthesis inhibition by NSAIDS will therefore reverse many of the clinical and biochemical abnormalities found in Bartter syndrome or phenotypically severe Gitelman syndrome (and EAST syndrome) [26].

4. Pendred Syndrome

Pendred syndrome is an autosomal recessive disorder resulting from biallelic mutations in *SLC26A4* which encodes Pendrin, a multi-functional anion transporter. Pendrin acts a chloride/bicarbonate exchanger in the cochlear, mediates iodide transport in the apical membrane of thyrocytes and as a chloride/bicarbonate exchanger in the apical membrane of beta-intercalated cells in the collecting duct (**Figure 3**). The resulting clinical picture is of sensorineural deafness, hypothyroidism, goitre and impaired bicarbonate secretion in states of metabolic alkalosis.

http://dx.doi.org/10.5772/intechopen.78724

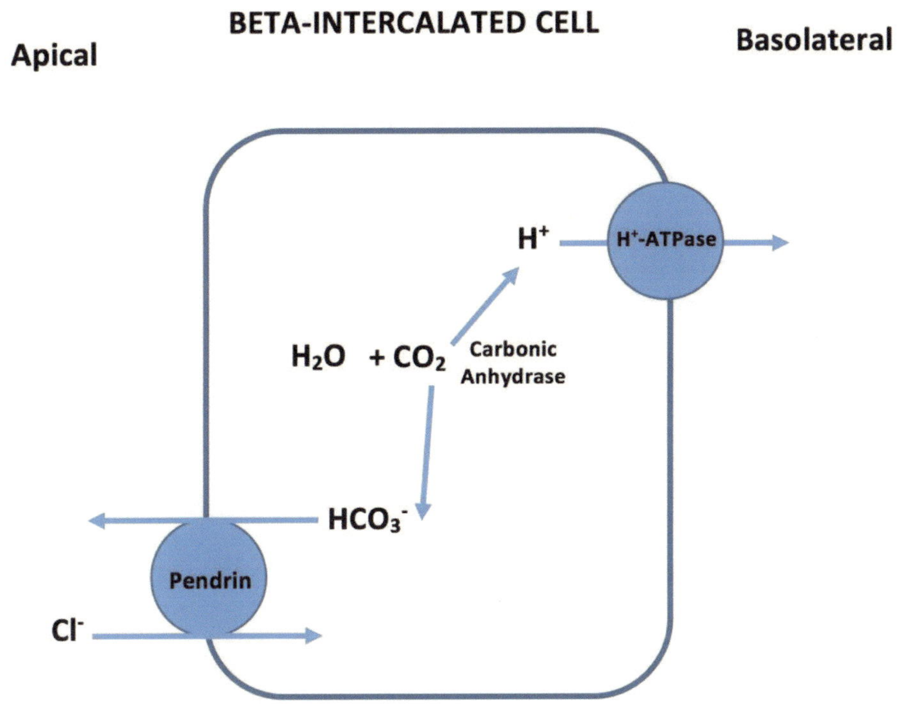

Figure 3. Pendrin expression in the intercalated cells of the kidney.

Failure of the compensatory mechanisms in alkalotic states such as those triggered by diuretics, including thiazides, can result in a life threatening metabolic alkalosis [27].

Pendrin is expressed on the apical membranes of type B intercalated cells (shown) as well as and non-A, non-B intercalated cells (not shown). Mutations in *SLC26A4*, which encodes Pendrin, lead to a failure of the kidney to secrete a bicarbonate load, which is generated from intracellular carbonic anhydrase type 2, leading towards a metabolic alkalosis.

4.1. Glucocorticoid remedial Aldosteronism

Glucocorticoid remediable aldosteronism (GRA) is an autosomal dominant inherited cause of hypertension and is one of three known forms of familial hyperaldosteronism. Normally, aldosterone synthesis occurs in the zona glomerulosa of the adrenal gland which intentionally lacks the 17-hydroxylase enzyme to synthesise cortisol. In GRA, aldosterone is synthesised in the ACTH-sensitive zona fasciculata. In the zona glomerulosa, the gene *CYP11B2* encodes aldosterone synthase which catalyses the conversion of deoxycorticosterone to corticosterone and 18-hydroxycorticosterone to aldosterone. In the zona fasciculata, *CYP11B1*, which encodes 11β-hydroxylase, catalyses the conversion of 11-deoxycortisol to cortisol. In GRA, there is a chimeric gene duplication that results from unequal crossing over of CYP11B1 and CYP11B2 resulting in ACTH-dependent activation of aldosterone synthase (rather than by the renin-angiotensin-aldosterone system) which causes a significant increase in 18-oxocortisol and

18-hydroxycortisol. As this reaction occurs in the zona fasciculate, the aldosterone secretion is not sensitive to potassium loading as it would be in a normal subject due to the consistent prolonged release of ACTH. Consequentially, you do not always get hypokalaemia with this condition in contrast to subjects with other forms of hyperaldosteronism. Hypertension typically develops before the age of 21 and significant hypokalaemia develops following thiazide diuretic administration due to its effect on increased distal tubular sodium delivery to aldosterone-sensitive potassium secretion site in the collecting duct. Although there is intra-family phenotypic variability with GRA, there is a strong prevalence of haemorrhagic stroke related to cerebral aneurysm which is even more prevalent than seen in autosomal dominant polycystic kidney disease [28, 29]. Subjects with GRA should subsequently have a cerebral MRA every 5 years from puberty. Genetic testing is now preferred to a dexamethasone suppression test and demonstration of elevated 18-oxocortisol and 18-hydroxycortisol [30]. Treatment comprises of ACTH suppression with glucocorticoids with careful attention to the growth retardation effects of over-treatment in paediatric subjects. This will restore normotension and normokalaemia. Alternatively, mineralocorticoid receptor antagonists such as spironolactone may be used [31].

4.2. Congenital adrenal hyperplasia

Over 95% of patients with congenital adrenal hyperplasia have defective conversion of 17-hydroxyprogesterone (17OHP) to 11-deoxycortisol. This is because of a mutation in the *CYP21A2* gene which encodes the enzyme 21-hydroxylase which is responsible for this conversion. CAH is an autosomal recessive disorder comprising two distinct types based on whether the condition is accompanied by salt wasting. Girls typically present with atypical genitalia (clitoral enlargement, urogenital sinus, labial fold fusion and genital orifice migration) but can present simply with severe salt wasting alone in the neonatal period. Boys typically present with severe salt wasting and do not manifest genital abnormalities until they reach an early onset puberty when they are toddlers. Phallic enlargement and hyperpigmentation can occur. CAH is diagnosed when the serum 17-hydroxyprogesterone concentration is elevated. Adrenal ultrasound has additional diagnostic value in the neonatal period revealing a lobulated surface, adrenal limb length greater than 4 mm and abnormal echogenicity. A prenatal diagnosis can be made by molecular analysis of *CYP21A2*. Treatment involves a glucocorticoid such as hydrocortisone to replace cortisol deficiency and hyperandrogenaemia and subsequent fertility difficulties. Mineralocorticoid replacement such as fludrocortisone is necessary to reverse salt wasting and volume depletion and testicular US surveillance from adolescence due to an increased risk of testicular adrenal rest tumours [32, 33].

4.3. Apparent mineralocorticoid excess

Mineralocorticoid receptors in the collecting duct bind aldosterone and cortisol with similar affinity. Cortisol is normally converted into its inactive form cortisone by the enzyme 11-beta-hydroxysteroid type 2 at sites of aldosterone activity to prevent competitive inhibition with aldosterone. In AME, a mutation in 11-beta-hydroxysteroid type 2 results in a reduction of cortisol conversion to cortisone and subsequently the mineralocorticoid receptor is activated

http://dx.doi.org/10.5772/intechopen.78724

by excess cortisol. AME is autosomal recessive and causes severe hypertension in children in addition to hypercalciuria, nephrocalcinosis and renal failure due to an unknown mechanism. Nephrogenic diabetes insipidus can also occur due to chronic hypokalaemia. Defects in *HSD11B2* are responsible for this condition, some mutations result only in partial inhibition of 11-beta hydroxysteroid 2 resulting in a less severe phenotype. There is rough genotypic-phenotypic correlation which includes the ratio of cortisol to cortisol metabolites which can be measured. Treatment for this condition aims at reducing endogenous cortisol production by dexamethasone or by blocking the mineralocorticoid receptor with spironolactone/eplerenone. ENaC blockade has similar success with less side effects, so it is reasonable to instead use amiloride or triamterene especially in men. If hypercalciuria is present then it is reasonable to use a thiazide to prevent nephrocalcinosis and subsequent renal impairment [34–36].

4.4. Liquorice ingestion and carbenoxolone

Liquorice (root of *Glycyrrhiza glabra*) is found in tobacco, snuff, foods, soft drinks, herbal medicine and teas in addition to its popular consumption as a confectionary item. Not all sweets contain the compound glycyrrhiza but instead are flavoured with alternative compounds to mimic liquorice so chronic ingestion should not cause the clinical picture of apparent mineralocorticoid excess. Glycyrrhiza inhibits 11-beta hydroxysteroid dehydrogenase which converts cortisol to cortisone. Carbenoxolone, a liquorice-like compound has the same effect [37].

4.5. Liddle syndrome

Liddle syndrome is a rare autosomal dominant disorder associated with a gain of function mutation in the epithelial sodium channel (ENaC) situated on the luminal membrane of principal cells in the collecting duct. In Liddle syndrome, ENaC function is increased which results in hypokalaemia and metabolic alkalosis. Increased activity of ENaC results in increased sodium reabsorption and potassium secretion and subsequent hypertension, hypokalaemia and metabolic alkalosis. Most patients present at a young age and not all have hypokalaemia but their potassium does run at lower range of normal.

Net sodium reabsorption occurs down a concentration gradient in principle cells via both ENaC on the luminal membrane and the Na–K–ATPase on the basolateral membrane. The greater net sodium reabsorption enhances potassium secretion through basolateral Na–K–ATPase and subsequent open luminal potassium channels.

Mutations in *SCNN1B* and *SCNN1G* which encode the beta and gamma subunits of ENaC cause Liddle syndrome. When volume expansion occurs there is failure to remove ENaC channels from the luminal membrane under the influence of low renin and aldosterone and the phenotype mimics a hyperaldosteronism state yet plasma and urine aldosterone levels are in fact reduced. Treatment involves potassium paring diuretics which directly block ENaC such as Amiloride or Triamterene. Spironolactone, which competes with aldosterone to bind to the mineralocorticoid receptor, would not be effective as increased ENaC activity in not mediated by aldosterone [38, 39].

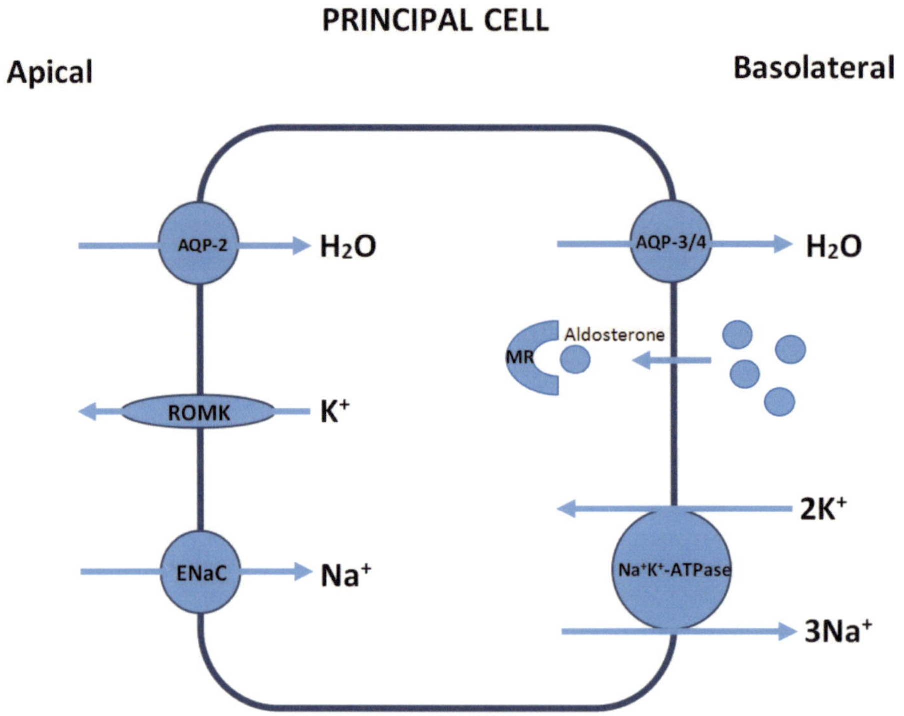

Figure 4. Salt transport in the principal cell.

4.6. Cortisol excess

Excess cortisol may allow stimulation of the mineralocorticoid receptor to leading to hypertension and a hypokalemic metabolic alkalosis. Causes include excess exogenous administration of glucocorticoids such as hydrocortisone or secondary to endogenous cortisol hypersecretion either by Cushing's syndrome or disease, ectopic ACTH production most commonly by small cell lung cancers or by a deoxycorticosterone-secreting tumour on the adrenal gland [2] (**Figure 4**).

Principal cells respond to a variety of stimuli to control Na^+ and K^+ transport. Aldosterone has the most pronounced effect. It acts through the mineralocorticoid receptor (MR) to increase surface expression of the epithelial sodium channel ENaC. Electrogenic Na^+ reabsorption via ENaC is balanced by K^+ secretion through ROMK and Cl^- reabsorption through multiple pathways (not shown). The driving force that sets the electrochemical gradient for principal cell Na^+ and K^+ transport is the basolateral Na^+–K^+–ATPase.

5. Reasons to suspect and inherited cause of alkalosis

Clinical features of a metabolic alkalosis include muscle cramps, weakness, arrhythmias and seizures. Some of these signs and symptoms may be related to alterations in ionised calcium

http://dx.doi.org/10.5772/intechopen.78724

(increased pH causes plasma proteins to bind calcium more avidly, thus lowering ionised calcium concentration). The associated hypokalaemia may also give rise to many of these symptoms. Inherited forms of alkalosis are secondary to a heterogeneous group of renal tubulopathies. Typical manifestations range from asymptomatic biochemical disturbances to severe salt wasting leading in early life and may be complicated by renal failure. The important clues to diagnosing an inherited cause of metabolic alkalosis include consistent electrolyte abnormalities (versus acquired changes in serum biochemistry), nephrocalcinosis, renal stone formation and renal impairment. Historical blood values are invaluable in this regard. A detailed family history is required to look for autosomal dominant and recessive patterns of disease. In children, failure to thrive, short stature, learning difficulties and rickets may also be evident. A history of early onset hypertension and a family history of stroke at a young age provides clues to look for inherited forms of hypertension including Liddle syndrome and GRA.

Individual syndromes may be distinguished by distinct biochemical profiles but modern day molecular genetics allows a more robust means to come to a firm diagnosis. A very similar biochemical picture to Bartter and Gitelman syndromes can be induced by diuretic use or abuse, laxative abuse and chronic liquorice ingestion. However, urinary chloride will be raised in Bartter and Gitelman syndromes (>20 mmol/L) whereas vomiting, gastric drainage, diuretics and post-hypercapnia will all have a low urinary chloride concentration (<10 mmol/L). Therefore, obtaining a careful drug and food history is important together with urine electrolyte analysis and diuretic screening to make certain that the cause is not an acquired one. The optimal treatment of a metabolic alkalosis clearly depends on identifying the underlying cause. Treatment of life-threatening alkalosis may involve control of ventilation (sedation, intubation and controlled hypoventilation). Historically, administration of HCl or ammonium chloride/arginine chloride has been advocated. These are not advocated. Control of ventilation and correction of volume status and improvement of renal haemodynamics is effective in cases of chloride loss. Haemodialysis may be used in extreme cases. Hypokalaemia should be corrected alongside the alkalosis. Treatment of Bartter and Gitelman syndrome, as detailed above, relies upon electrolyte replacement, attempts at disrupting the renal production of renin with NSAIDs and blocking the effects of excess mineralocorticoids with spironolactone, eplerenone and amiloride. Treatment of Liddle syndrome relies on sodium restriction and potassium-sparing diuretics which block ENaC and allow the correction of blood pressure, hypokalaemia and metabolic alkalosis.

6. Conclusions

A systemic metabolic alkalosis is an important electrolyte disturbance which can have significant sequelae including neuromuscular irritability, tetany and cardiac rhythm disturbances. Hypokalaemia is a frequent accompanying electrolyte abnormality. Numerous inherited tubulopathies can cause this clinical and biochemical picture and acquired causes may mimic these. Molecular genetic testing allows a precise diagnosis and appropriate management to be given to patients with inherited salt wasting alkaloses.

Author details

Holly Mabillard and John A. Sayer*

*Address all correspondence to: john.sayer@ncl.ac.uk

Institute of Genetic Medicine, Newcastle University, Newcastle Upon Tyne, United Kingdom

References

[1] Hamm L, Nakhoul N, Hering-Smith KS. Acid Base Homeostasis. Clinical Journal of the American Society of Nephrology. 2015;**10**(12):2232-2242

[2] Johnson R, Feehally J, Floege J. Comprehensive Clinical Nephrology. Vol. 5e. Elsevier; 2014

[3] Palmer BF, Alpern RJ. Metabolic alkalosis. Journal of the American Society of Nephrology. 1997;**8**(9):1462

[4] Khanna A, Kurtzman NA. Metabolic alkalosis. Journal of Nephrology. 2006;**19**:S86

[5] Galla JH. Metabolic alkalosis. Journal of the American Society of Nephrology. 2000;**11**(2):369

[6] Wile D. Diuretics: A review. Annals of Clinical Biochemistry: International Journal of Laboratory Medicine. 2012;**49**(5):419-431

[7] Greenberg A. Diuretic complications. The American Journal of the Medical Sciences. 2000; **319**(1):10-24

[8] Polak A, Haynie GD, Hays RM, Schwartz WB. Effects of chronic hypercapnia on electrolyte and acid-base equilibrium. Journal of Clinical Investigation. 1961;**40**:1223

[9] Schwartz WB, van Ypersele de Strihou C, Kassirer JP. Role of anions in metabolic alkalosis and potassium deficiency. New England Journal of Medicine. 1968;**279**:630-639

[10] Kurtz I. Molecular pathogenesis of Bartter's and Gitelman's syndromes. Kidney International. 1998;**54**:1396

[11] Stein JH. The pathogenetic spectrum of Bartter's syndrome. Kidney International. 1985;**28**:85

[12] Simon DB, Nelson-Williams C, Bia MJ, et al. Gitelman's variant of Bartter's syndrome, inherited hypokalaemic alkalosis, is caused by mutations in the thiazide-sensitive Na-Cl cotransporter. Nature Genetics. 1996;**12**:24

[13] Waldegger S, Jentsch TJ. From tonus to tonicity: Physiology of CLC chloride channels. Journal of the American Society of Nephrology. 2000;**11**:1331

[14] Zelikovic I. Hypokalaemic salt-losing tubulopathies: An evolving story. Nephrology, Dialysis, Transplantation. 2003;**18**:1696

[15] Brochard K, Boyer O, Blanchard A, et al. Phenotype-genotype correlation in antenatal and neonatal variants of Bartter syndrome. Nephrology, Dialysis, Transplantation. 2009; **24**:1455

[16] Andrini O, Keck M, Briones R, et al. ClC-K chloride channels: Emerging pathophysiology of Bartter syndrome type 3. American Journal of Physiology. Renal Physiology. 2015; **308**:F1324

[17] Birkenhäger R, Otto E, Schürmann MJ, et al. Mutation of BSND causes Bartter syndrome with sensorineural deafness and kidney failure. Nature Genetics. 2001;**29**:310

[18] Watanabe S, Fukumoto S, Chang H, et al. Association between activating mutations of calcium-sensing receptor and Bartter's syndrome. Lancet. 2002;**360**:692

[19] Laghmani K. Polyhydramnios, transient antenatal Bartter's syndrome, and MAGED2 mutations. New England Journal of Medicine. 2016;**374**(19):1853-1863

[20] Jeck N, Konrad M, Peters M, et al. Mutations in the chloride channel gene CLCNKB leading to a mixed Bartter-Gitelman phenotype. Paediatric Research. 2000;**48**(6):754-758

[21] Gitelman HJ, Graham JB, Welt LG. A new familial disorder characterized by hypokalaemia and hypomagnesaemia. Transactions of the Association of American Physicians. 1966;**79**:221-235

[22] Vargas-Poussou R, Dahan K, Kahila D, et al. Spectrum of mutations in Gitelman syndrome. Journal of the American Society of Nephrology. 2011;**22**(4):693-703

[23] Bockenhauer D, Feather S, Stanescu HC, et al. Epilepsy, ataxia, sensorineural deafness, tubulopathy, and KCNJ10 mutations. New England Journal of Medicine. 2009;**360**(19): 1960-1970

[24] Scholl UI, Choi M, Liu T, et al. Seizures, sensorineural deafness, ataxia, mental retardation, and electrolyte imbalance (SeSAME syndrome) caused by mutations in KCNJ10. Proceedings of the National Academy of Sciences of the United States of America. 2009;**14**:5842-5847

[25] Kömhoff M, Reinalter SC, Gröne HJ, Seyberth HW. Induction of microsomal prostaglandin E2 synthase in the macula densa in children with hypokalemic salt-losing tubulopathies. Pediatric Research. 2004;**55**:261

[26] Blanchard A, Vargas-Poussou R, Vallet M, et al. Indomethacin, amiloride, or eplerenone for treating hypokalemia in Gitelman syndrome. ournal of the American Society of Nephrology. 2015;**26**:468

[27] Kandasamy N et al. Life-threatening metabolic alkalosis in Pendred syndrome. European Journal of Endocrinology. 2011;**165**(1):167-170

[28] McMahon GT, Dluhy RG. Glucocorticoid-remediable aldosteronism. Cardiology in Review. 2004;**12**:44

[29] Rich GM, Ulick S, Cook S, et al. Glucocorticoid-remediable aldosteronism in a large kindred: Clinical spectrum and diagnosis using a characteristic biochemical phenotype. Annals of Internal Medicine. 1992;**116**:813

[30] Jonsson JR, Klemm SA, Tunny TJ, et al. A new genetic test for familial hyperaldosteronism type I aids in the detection of curable hypertension. Biochemical and Biophysical Research Communications. 1995;**207**:565

[31] Funder JW, Carey RM, Mantero F, et al. The management of primary aldosteronism: Case detection, diagnosis, and treatment: An Endocrine Society Clinical Practice Guideline. The Journal of Clinical Endocrinology and Metabolism. 2016;**101**:1889

[32] Merke DP, Bornstein SR. Congenital adrenal hyperplasia. Lancet. 2005;**365**:2125

[33] Joint LWPES/ESPE CAH Working Group. Consensus statement on 21-hydroxylase deficiency from the Lawson Wilkins Pediatric Endocrine Society and the European Society for Paediatric Endocrinology. The Journal of Clinical Endocrinology and Metabolism. 2002;**87**:4048

[34] Funder JW. Apparent mineralocorticoid excess. The Journal of Steroid Biochemistry and Molecular Biology. 2017;**165**:151

[35] Funder JW. 11 beta-hydroxysteroid dehydrogenase: New answers, new questions. European Journal of Endocrinology. 1996;**134**:267

[36] Mune T, Rogerson FM, Nikkilä H, et al. Human hypertension caused by mutations in the kidney isozyme of 11 beta-hydroxysteroid dehydrogenase. Nature Genetics. 1995;**10**:394

[37] Farese RV, Biglieri EG, Shackleton CH, et al. Licorice-induced hypermineralocorticoidism. The New England Journal of Medicine. 1991;**325**:1223

[38] Botero-Velez M, Curtis JJ, Warnock DG. Brief report: Liddle's syndrome revisited—A disorder of sodium reabsorption in the distal tubule. The New England Journal of Medicine. 1994;**330**:178

[39] Snyder PM, Price MP, McDonald FJ, et al. Mechanism by which Liddle's syndrome mutations increase activity of a human epithelial Na^+ channel. Cell. 1995;**83**:969

Chapter 4

Bartter and Gitelman Syndromes

Caius Mihai Breazu, Adrian Bartos and Dana Bartos

Additional information is available at the end of the chapter

http://dx.doi.org/10.5772/intechopen.81745

Abstract

Bartter and Gitelman syndromes are rare genetic disorders in which there are specific defects in kidney function, characterized by metabolic alkalosis, hypokalemia, hyperreninemia, and hyperaldosteronism, with or without hypomagnesemia. Blood pressure is normal or low in these patients. Positive diagnosis is one of the exclusions, and the difference between the two syndromes is based on urine calcium levels. Medication has to be taken lifelong. Renal transplantation can correct the transport defect in Bartter and Gitelman syndromes. The symptoms and severity vary from one person to another and can range from mild to severe. Age of onset of overt symptoms can range from before birth to adulthood.

Keywords: Bartter syndrome, genes, mutations, electrolyte imbalances

1. Introduction

Bartter syndrome, originally described by Bartter and colleagues in 1962 [1], represents an autosomal recessive renal tubular disorder characterized by hypokalemia and metabolic alkalosis. In addition, patients have hyperreninemia and hyperplasia of the juxtaglomerular apparatus (the source of renin in the kidney) and secondary hyperaldosteronism [2]. The underlying renal abnormality results in excessive urinary losses of sodium, chloride, and potassium.

2. Etiology

Bartter and Gitelman syndromes are caused by the alteration of a carrier involved in sodium chloride (NaCl) reabsorption. This transporter is located in the thick ascending limb of the loop of Henle in Bartter syndrome and distal convoluted tubule in Gitelman syndrome [3].

Bartter syndrome subtype	Genetic defect	Clinical syndrome
Type I	SLC12A1 (NKCC2)	Antenatal Bartter syndrome
Type II	KCNJ1 (ROMK)	Antenatal Bartter syndrome
Type III	CLCKB	Classic Bartter syndrome
Type IV	BSND	Antenatal Bartter syndrome with congenital hearing loss
Type IV B	CLCNKA CLCNKB	Antenatal Bartter syndrome with congenital hearing loss
Type V	CaSR	Bartter syndrome with hypocalcaemia
Gitelman syndrome	SLC12A3 (NCCT)	Gitelman syndrome

Table 1. Bartter syndrome subtypes.

Bartter syndrome results from defective transepithelial transport of NaCl in the thick ascending loop or the distal convoluted tubule.

- Transepithelial Cl transport in the thick ascending loop depends on coordinated interplay between the luminal, bumetanide-sensitive, Na-K-2Cl co-transporter (NKCC2), the luminal, K channel (ROMK), the basolateral Cl channel (CIC-Kb), as well as other co-transporters and channels [4].
- Chloride transport in the distal convoluted tubule occurs primarily via the luminal, thiazide-sensitive NaCl co-transporter [4].

There are six subtypes of Bartter syndrome (I, II, III, IV, IVB, and V), each corresponding to a genetic defect (**Table 1**).

Types I through IV—the severity and clinical presentation of Bartter syndrome varies with each type:

- Types I and II are the most severe disorders. They are characterized by polyhydramnios during pregnancy and premature birth. Those who survive infancy develop hypokalemia, metabolic alkalosis, polyuria, and hypercalciuria. Neonates with type II mutations that reduce activity of the renal outer medullary potassium channel (ROMK) often initially develop hyperkalemia [4]. However, as they mature, other potassium channels become active and contribute to the development of hypokalemia. Nephrocalcinosis is common in patients with these mutations and probably contributes to the late development of kidney dysfunction and, rarely, end-stage renal disease [5].
- The classic form of Bartter syndrome, type III, is less severe and presents later in life with hypokalemia, metabolic alkalosis, and hypercalciuria. The reduced severity of type III Bartter syndrome may be due to redundancy of chloride channels in the cells of the thick ascending limb. Loss of ClC-Kb activity causes the disease, but coexistent ClC-Ka activity may ameliorate the process. Some patients with ClC-Kb mutations usually have classic Bartter

http://dx.doi.org/10.5772/intechopen.81745

syndrome that occurs in infancy or early childhood. It is characterized by hypomagnesemia, hypocalciuria (not hypercalciuria), and unresponsiveness to thiazide rather than loop diuretics [6, 7]. This may be seen because ClC-Kb participates in chloride reabsorption along the distal convoluted tubule and connecting tubule, as well as the thick ascending limb [8]. Many of the mutations that cause Bartter syndrome type III destabilize channel structure, induce ClC-Kb retention within the endoplasmic reticulum, and accelerate channel degradation [6].

- Types IV and IVb have combined defects that involve both the ClC-Ka and ClC-Kb channels and cause severe disease, generally with antenatal presentation and congenital hearing loss. These two chloride channels are critical for normal ion transport in the stria vascularis of the inner ear and are vital to establish normal endocochlear potential differences [9–14]. Because of redundancy of function in the ear, hearing loss requires defects to exist in both ClC-Ka and ClC-Kb. This double defect can occur via at least two mechanisms:
    - As discussed above, the Barttin subunit is an important component of both channels. Thus, a single defect that affects the Barttin subunit reduces the function of both channels (type IV) [9–13]. Hereditary defect in Barttin leads to antenatal Bartter syndrome associated with sensorineural deafness and renal failure.
    - The other mechanism involves double mutations, which reduce the function of both ClC-Ka and ClC-Kb and thereby produce a phenotype similar to the Barttin type IV defect. This is generally called Bartter type IVb [15]. Although some have called this variant "Bartter type V disease," the designation "type V Bartter disease" is most commonly used to describe a gain-of-function mutation in CaSR.
- Type V, usually called autosomal dominant hypocalcemia or autosomal dominant hypoparathyroidism, is due to a gain-of-function mutation in CaSR, encoding the calcium-sensing receptor (CaSR) [16, 17]. In the parathyroid gland, this results in a downward "resetting" of the normal range for serum calcium. As a result, a lower-than-normal serum calcium concentration inhibits parathyroid hormone release, resulting in hypocalcemia.

The tubular defect found in Bartter syndrome is the same as in the chronic ingestion of loop diuretics, while in Gitelman syndrome, it is the same as in the chronic ingestion of thiazide diuretics. In both the syndromes, elevated salt removal will lead to volume depletion and activation of the renin-angiotensin-aldosterone system. The association of secondary hyperaldosteronism with increasing concentration of NaCl at the distal level leads to increased potassium and hydrogen secretion in collecting tubule and distal convoluted tubule, resulting in hypopotassemia and metabolic alkalosis.

The volume depletion explains why patients with Bartter or Gitelman syndrome have lower blood pressure than general population. In addition, in patients with Bartter syndrome, another possible cause of this phenomenon is increased prostaglandin renal clearance with a vasodilator effect [4]. Because urine dilution requires good functioning of the ascending portion of the loop of Henle and the distal convoluted tubule, Bartter and Gitelman syndromes have a low urine dilution capacity [1].

There are also a number of distinct traits between the two syndromes caused by the different site of the NaCl reabsorption abnormality. Thus, patients with Bartter syndrome have a poor response to the action of loop diuretics, while patients with Gitelman syndrome have a lower response to thiazide diuretics [4].

Calciuresis is normal or increased in Bartter syndrome, similar to loop diuretic effect. On the contrary, calciuresis is low in Gitelman syndrome, as in the use of thiazide diuretics.

3. Prevalence

Gitelman syndrome is a much more common disease than Bartter syndrome [18, 19]. For Gitelman syndrome, a prevalence of 1:40,000 is reported, while Bartter syndrome is less common in the population (1:1,000,000) [18]. The lower prevalence of Bartter syndrome in the population may be due at least in part to prenatal or neonatal death resulting from the disorder before it could be diagnosed [18].

4. Clinical manifestation

Table 2 summarizes the similar and distinct clinical features in Bartter and Gitelman syndromes. In both the syndromes, clinical manifestations are less pronounced in heterozygotes.

Bartter syndrome I, II, IV, and IVB subtypes are most often severe early-onset disease, while subtypes III and V are lighter forms of late-onset disease. However, the correlation between the underlying genetic defect and the clinical phenotype is not absolute.

Subtypes I and II begin antenatally with polyhydramnios and prematurity. Patients who survive infancy develop hypokalemia, metabolic alkalosis, polyuria, and hypercalciuria.

Subtype III is the classic form of Bartter syndrome, starting later than the first subtypes with hypokalemia, metabolic alkalosis, and hypercalciuria. During the course of the disease, this subtype may be associated with proteinuria and renal failure.

Bartter syndrome	Gitelman syndrome
It usually occurs in childhood	It usually occurs in adolescents and adults
Growth retardation present	Growth retardation absent
Normal or low blood pressure	Normal or low blood pressure
Dehydration present	Dehydration absent
Hypokalemic metabolic alkalosis	Hypokalemic metabolic alkalosis
Polyuria and polydipsia present	Polyuria and polydipsia absent
Normocalciuria or hypercalciuria	Hypocalciuria
Maternal polyhydramnios common	Maternal polyhydramnios absent
Normal or slightly low magnesium	Hypomagnesemia

Table 2. Clinical features of Bartter and Gitelman syndromes.

Subtypes IV and IVB usually begin antenatally and should be associated with neurosensory deafness, as the underlying genetic defect affects both NaCl conveying ion channels in the kidney and inner ear.

Subtype V is also known as autosomal-dominant hypocalcaemia or autosomal-dominant hypoparathyroidism. In this case, the underlying genetic defect leads to a "reset" of the normal serum calcium level. Thus, a lower value than normal can inhibit the secretion of parathyroid hormone, leading to hypocalcemia.

5. Differential diagnosis

- Other causes of unexplained hypokalemia and metabolic alkalosis
  - Vomiting/diarrhea
  - Diuretic abuse (**Figure 1**)

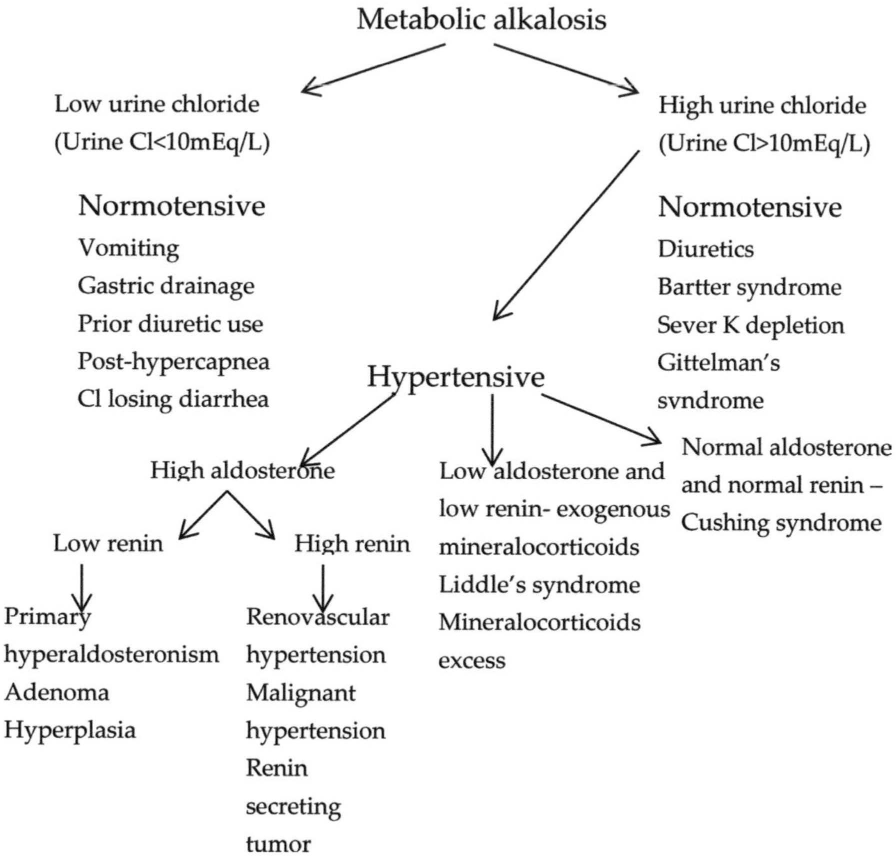

Figure 1. Differential diagnostic of metabolic alkalosis [20].

6. Laboratory studies

- Serum potassium levels—low in all forms of Bartter syndrome
- Serum calcium levels—normal to low
- Serum magnesium levels—low or normal in Bartter syndrome, low in Gitelman syndrome
- Aldosterone levels—elevated
- Urinary potassium levels—elevated
- Urinary aldosterone levels—high
- Urinary chloride levels—high

7. Treatment

The tubular defects in Bartter syndrome cannot be corrected (except by renal transplantation). Thus, treatment is aimed at minimizing the effects of secondary increases in renin, aldosterone, and, in some patients, prostaglandins, as well as correcting the volume deficit and electrolyte abnormalities. There is no consensus on the best treatment for Gitelman syndrome, and magnesium and potassium supplements are usually given.

7.1. NSAIDs and drugs that block distal convoluted tubule sodium-potassium exchange

Nonsteroidal anti-inflammatory drugs (NSAIDs) are an essential component of therapy and can ameliorate many of the abnormalities. The defect in the thick ascending limb of the loop of Henle function in Bartter syndrome often increases renal prostaglandin E2 (PGE2) production. This also occurs with therapeutic loop diuretic use. Markedly increased PGE2 is common in patients with Bartter syndrome types I, II, IV, and IVb.

Indomethacin and celecoxib have been used; there are no clear advantages with either drug [21]. However, careful monitoring is required since NSAIDs can have significant adverse effects including renal and gastrointestinal toxicity.

In addition to an NSAID, a drug that blocks distal convoluted tubule sodium-potassium exchange, such as spironolactone, eplerenone, or amiloride, is usually administered, frequently in higher-than-usual doses (up to 300, 150, and 40 mg/day, respectively). This regimen can raise the serum potassium, reverse the metabolic alkalosis, and partially correct the hypomagnesemia [21, 22]. Among patients with hypokalemia due to potassium wasting of any cause, drugs blocking distal sodium-potassium exchange are typically more effective and better tolerated than potassium supplementation alone.

7.2. Angiotensin-converting enzyme inhibitors

Angiotensin-converting enzyme (ACE) inhibitors reduce the production of angiotensin II and aldosterone and may be a useful adjunctive therapy [23, 24].

Angiotensin receptor blockers (ARBs) should have similar efficacy but have not been well studied in these patients. ACE inhibitors will also reduce proteinuria in these patients when it exists [25].

7.3. Potassium and magnesium supplementation

Most patients require oral potassium and magnesium supplementation since therapy with NSAIDs and drugs that block distal convoluted tubule sodium-potassium exchange is often incompletely effective [26]. However, the restoration of normal serum potassium and magnesium concentrations is often difficult to achieve for one or more of the following reasons:

- Blocking potassium secretion in the cortical collecting tubule with a drug that inhibits sodium-potassium exchange with or without an ACE inhibitor in patients with Bartter syndrome will not reverse the primary defect.
- Hypomagnesemia can contribute to urinary potassium loss.
- When hypokalemia and/or hypomagnesemia are due to urinary wasting, potassium or magnesium supplementation has limited efficacy. As the serum potassium and/or magnesium falls in the untreated patient, the antikaliuretic effect of hypokalemia and the antimagnesiuretic effect of hypomagnesemia gradually reduce potassium and magnesium excretion until a new steady state is attained in which intake and urinary excretion are similar and potassium and magnesium concentrations stabilize at a lower-than-normal level.

The rise in serum concentrations following the administration of potassium and magnesium supplements will reduce the stimulus to potassium and magnesium retention. As a result, most of the administered potassium or magnesium will be excreted in the urine. High doses, which are often difficult to tolerate (e.g., diarrhea with magnesium), are required to achieve a substantial elevation in serum potassium or magnesium. Similar considerations apply to hypokalemia and hypomagnesemia due to other causes of urinary wasting of these cations.

7.4. Renal transplantation

Renal transplantation corrects the transport abnormalities in Gitelman and Bartter syndromes, and recurrent disease in the transplant has not been described. Renal transplantation has been performed in rare patients who developed end-stage renal disease due to coexisting renal disease or the effects of chronic volume depletion, electrolyte abnormalities, drug-related side effects, and/or nephrocalcinosis [27, 28]. In addition, successful preemptive bilateral nephrectomy and renal transplantation have been performed in two patients with severe neonatal Bartter syndrome [28].

Acknowledgements

Caius Breazu is the coordinator of this chapter.

Author details

Caius Mihai Breazu[1,3]*, Adrian Bartos[2] and Dana Bartos[1,2]

*Address all correspondence to: csbreazu@yahoo.com

1 Surgery Department, Regional Institute of Gastroenterology and Hepatology "Prof Dr. Octavian Fodor", Cluj-Napoca, Romania

2 Anatomy and Embriology Department, UMF "Iuliu Hațieganu", Cluj-Napoca, Romania

3 Anesthesia and Intensive care Department, UMF "Iuliu Hațieganu", Cluj-Napoca, Romania

References

[1] Bartter FC, Pronove P, Gill JR. Hyperplasia of the juxtaglomerular complex with hyperaldosteronism and hypokalemic alkalosis. The American Journal of Medicine. 1962;**33**:811-828

[2] Bokhari SRA, Mansur A. Bartter Syndrome. StatPearls Publishing; 2007

[3] Fremont OT, Chan JC. Understanding Bartter syndrome and Gitelman syndrome. World Journal of Pediatrics. 2012;**8**(1):25-30

[4] Finer G, Shalev H, Birk OS, et al. Transient neonatal hyperkalemia in the antenatal (ROMK defective) Bartter syndrome. The Journal of Pediatrics. 2003;**142**:318

[5] Brochard K, Boyer O, Blanchard A, et al. Phenotype-genotype correlation in antenatal and neonatal variants of Bartter syndrome. Nephrology, Dialysis, Transplantation. 2009;**24**:1455

[6] Andrini O, Keck M, Briones R, et al. ClC-K chloride channels: Emerging pathophysiology of Bartter syndrome type 3. American Journal of Physiology. Renal Physiology. 2015;**308**:F1324

[7] Nozu K, Iijima K, Kanda K, et al. The pharmacological characteristics of molecular-based inherited salt-losing tubulopathies. The Journal of Clinical Endocrinology and Metabolism. 2010;**95**:E511

[8] Zaika O, Tomilin V, Mamenko M, et al. New perspective of ClC-Kb/2 Cl-channel physiology in the distal renal tubule. American Journal of Physiology. Renal Physiology. 2016;**310**:F923

[9] Birkenhäger R, Otto E, Schürmann MJ, et al. Mutation of BSND causes Bartter syndrome with sensorineural deafness and kidney failure. Nature Genetics. 2001;**29**:310

[10] Estévez R, Boettger T, Stein V, et al. Barttin is a Cl− channel beta-subunit crucial for renal Cl− reabsorption and inner ear K+ secretion. Nature. 2001;**414**:558

[11] Izzedine H, Tankere F, Launay-Vacher V, Deray G. Ear and kidney syndromes: Molecular versus clinical approach. Kidney International. 2004;**65**:369

[12] Kobayashi K, Uchida S, Okamura HO, et al. Human CLC-KB gene promoter drives the EGFP expression in the specific distal nephron segments and inner ear. Journal of the American Society of Nephrology. 2002;**13**:1992

[13] Janssen AG, Scholl U, Domeyer C, et al. Disease-causing dysfunctions of barttin in Bartter syndrome type IV. Journal of the American Society of Nephrology. 2009;**20**:145

[14] Kontorinis G, Giesemann AM, Iliodromiti Z, et al. Treating hearing loss in patients with infantile Bartter syndrome. Laryngoscope. 2012;**122**:2524

[15] Schlingmann KP, Konrad M, Jeck N, et al. Salt wasting and deafness resulting from mutations in two chloride channels. The New England Journal of Medicine. 2004;**350**:1314

[16] Hebert SC. Extracellular calcium-sensing receptor: Implications for calcium and magnesium handling in the kidney. Kidney International. 1996;**50**:2129

[17] Watanabe S, Fukumoto S, Chang H, et al. Association between activating mutations of calcium-sensing receptor and Bartter's syndrome. Lancet. 2002;**360**:692

[18] Ji W, Foo JN, O'Roak BJ, et al. Rare independent mutations in renal salt handling genes contribute to blood pressure variation. Nature Genetics. 2008;**40**:592

[19] Gladziwa U, Schwarz R, Gitter AH, et al. Chronic hypokalaemia of adults: Gitelman's syndrome is frequent but classical Bartter's syndrome is rare. Nephrology, Dialysis, Transplantation. 1995;**10**:1607

[20] Passariello A, Maddalena Y, Malamisura M, Aragione N, et al. Metabolic alkalosis resulting from a congenital duodenal diaphragm. Journal of Neonatal Surgery [S.l.]. Oct. 2014;**3**(4):48. ISSN: 2226-0439

[21] Blanchard A, Vargas-Poussou R, Vallet M, et al. Indomethacin, amiloride, or eplerenone for treating hypokalemia in Gitelman syndrome. Journal of the American Society of Nephrology. 2015;**26**:468

[22] Griffing GT, Komanicky P, Aurecchia SA, et al. Amiloride in Bartter's syndrome. Clinical Pharmacology and Therapeutics. 1982;**31**:713

[23] Hené RJ, Koomans HA, Dorhout Mees EJ, et al. Correction of hypokalemia in Bartter's syndrome by enalapril. American Journal of Kidney Diseases. 1987;**9**:200

[24] Morales JM, Ruilope LM, Praga M, et al. Long-term enalapril therapy in Bartter's syndrome. Nephron. 1988;**48**:327

[25] Nascimento CL, Garcia CL, Schvartsman BG, Vaisbich MH. Treatment of Bartter syndrome. Unsolved issue. Jornal de Pediatria. 2014;**90**:512

[26] Blanchard A, Bockenhauer D, Bolignano D, et al. Gitelman syndrome: Consensus and guidance from a kidney disease: Improving global outcomes (KDIGO) controversies conference. Kidney International. 2017;**91**:24

[27] Calò LA, Marchini F, Davis PA, et al. Kidney transplant in Gitelman's syndrome. Report of the first case. Journal of Nephrology. 2003;**16**:144

[28] Chaudhuri A, Salvatierra O Jr, Alexander SR, Sarwal MM. Option of pre-emptive nephrectomy and renal transplantation for Bartter's syndrome. Pediatric Transplantation. 2006;**10**:266

Chapter 5

Calcium, Phosphate and Magnesium Disorders

Vanessa Heron

Additional information is available at the end of the chapter

http://dx.doi.org/10.5772/intechopen.81173

Abstract

Calcium, phosphate and magnesium are essential for human function and life. Each electrolyte is readily found in the human diet, and homeostasis is tightly regulated by the intestine, kidney and bone as well as other critical hormones, receptors and transporters. Disturbance to this balance can result in symptomatic disease and life-threatening manifestations. Calcium and phosphate are particularly co-dependent with disruption to the balance of one often influencing the other. It is important that clinicians have a thorough understanding of the mechanisms underplaying the homeostasis of each electrolyte as they have implications for prevention and management of disease. This chapter aims to outline the importance of calcium, phosphate and magnesium; the regulation of each electrolyte and the consequences of imbalance.

Keywords: calcium, magnesium, phosphate, parathyroid hormone, fibroblast growth factor, vitamin D, hypercalcaemia, hypocalcaemia, hyperphosphataemia, hypophosphataemia, hypermagnesaemia, hypomagnesaemia

1. Introduction

Calcium, phosphate and magnesium are electrolytes essential to human function and life. The balance of each electrolyte is reliant on the interplay between the gastrointestinal tract, kidney and bone. Other hormones, receptors and transporters are also integral to calcium, phosphate and magnesium homeostasis, influencing the actions of the intestine, kidney and bone. This chapter will outline the importance of calcium, phosphate and magnesium, the mechanisms for regulation and the consequences of imbalance.

2. Calcium

2.1. The importance of calcium

The human body contains 1–2 kg of the divalent cation calcium. Greater than 99% of calcium is stored in bone, and this provides structure for the human skeleton. The remaining calcium is stored in the intracellular and extracellular space. Beyond its structural importance, calcium plays a role in functions including intracellular signalling, neuromuscular transmission, muscular function, endocrinological function, coagulation and intercellular adhesion [1].

Calcium homeostasis is maintained through a delicate relationship between organs, including the kidneys, intestine, parathyroid glands, and bone. This is mediated by hormones such as parathyroid hormone (PTH), vitamin D3 (cholecalciferol), calcitriol (1,25-dihydroxycholecalciferol), fibroblast growth factor 23 (FGF23) and klotho [2].

2.2. Dietary calcium

Calcium accumulation commences in the third trimester of pregnancy and increases during childhood, adolescence and into early adulthood, at which time calcium storage peaks. The net balance of calcium is determined by the difference between calcium intake and calcium loss.

Throughout childhood and early adulthood, a positive calcium balance is required for bone growth. In this age group, as little as 500 mg of dietary calcium intake results in a positive calcium balance and the efficiency of intestinal calcium absorption can accommodate for the amount of calcium intake [3]. Between 25 and 35 years of age, when bone growth is complete, the net calcium balance should be neutral. With ageing, bone mass decreases due to net resorption of bone at a rate of less than 1–2% per year [4]. However, menopause leads to a negative balance because of difficulties with intestinal absorption attributed to by oestrogen deficiency [2]. Postmenopausal women require 1200 mg of dietary calcium to achieve a positive calcium balance [3, 5].

2.3. Physiology of calcium

Calcium exists in the human body stored as bone (calcium hydroxyapatite) and is otherwise found in the extracellular or intracellular space. One percent of skeletal calcium can be exchanged freely with the extracellular space via the osteoblastic and osteoclastic actions of bone [1, 4]. Forty-eight percent of serum calcium is ionised, and this is its physiologically active state. Forty-six percent is bound to protein, and 7% forms a complex with phosphate, citrate, sulphate, bicarbonate or other anions [1, 2].

Measurement of the plasma calcium is a reflection of the calcium bound to proteins such as albumin and immunoglobulin. The normal range is 2.1–2.6 mmol/L (8.5–10.5 mg/dL) [2]. For every 1 g/dL reduction in the serum albumin, serum calcium decreases by 0.8 mg/dL. Similarly, a 1 g/dL reduction in serum globulin results in serum calcium decreasing by 0.12 mg/dL [1]. While these formulas exist to calculate a corrected calcium level, they have been found to have poor sensitivity and specificity in detecting true hypocalcaemia or hypercalcaemia. Ionised calcium levels are felt to be a more accurate representation of the physiologically active level [2].

In the context of acute metabolic alkalosis, hydrogen ions dissociate from albumin. This subsequently allows albumin to bind more calcium, decreasing the circulating ionised calcium. Ionised calcium levels will fall by 0.12 mg/dL for each change in pH of 0.1 [1].

Extracellular calcium homeostasis is mediated by the gastrointestinal system, kidneys and bone.

2.3.1. Renal handling of calcium

Around 8–10 g of ionised calcium is filtered by the kidneys each day. Of this, around 100–200 mg (2–3% of total filtered calcium) is excreted in the urine [1, 3, 4].

Around 60–70% of calcium is reabsorbed in the proximal convoluted tubule (PCT). This mainly occurs passively via a transepithelial electrochemical gradient established by the reabsorption of sodium and water. A small amount of calcium is reabsorbed by active calcium transport. The process of reabsorption is controlled by PTH and calcitonin [1].

There is no calcium reabsorption in the thin loop of Henle, but a further 20% of calcium is reabsorbed in the thick ascending loop of Henle (TALH). This is predominately mediated by paracellular transport, although some transcellular movement occurs. The apical Na-K-2Cl (NKCC2) transporter and the renal outer medullary potassium channel (ROMK) produce a lumen-positive transepithelial gradient for paracellular cation transport, which is caused by a back flux of potassium into the lumen [6, 7]. This consequently causes paracellular calcium reabsorption as demonstrated in **Figure 1** [1, 8]. It also contributes to the reabsorption of other cations such as magnesium and sodium.

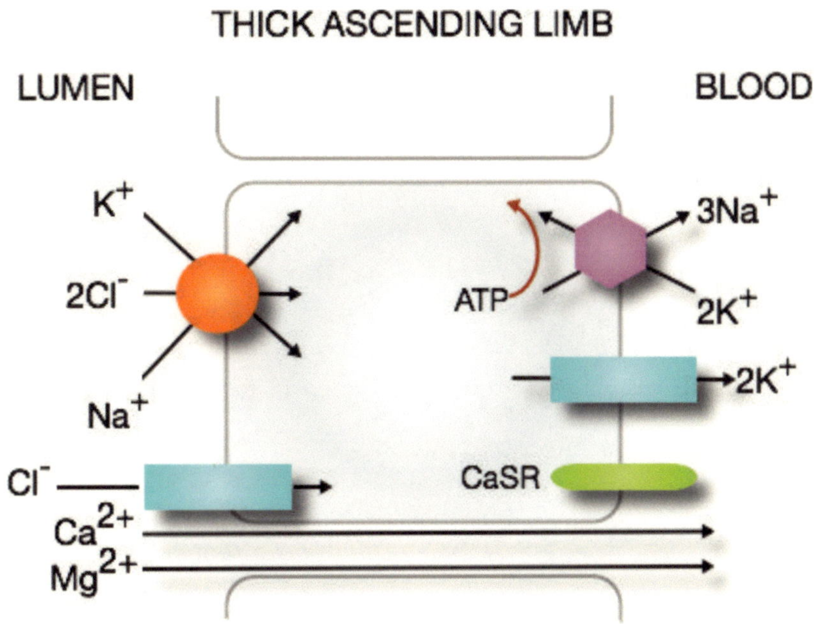

Figure 1. Calcium reabsorption at the thick ascending limb of the loop of Henle. The apical Na-K-2Cl transporter and the renal outer medullary potassium channel are responsible for creating a transepithelial gradient, which drives paracellular calcium transport [1]

The calcium-sensing receptor (CaSR) on the basolateral membrane of the TALH is a G-protein-coupled receptor. It is made up of a large extracellular and cytoplasmic domain [2]. Downregulation of the CaSR increases calcium permeability, while activation impedes permeability. The CaSR inhibits the ROMK channel in the presence of hypercalcaemia, leading to a reduction in paracellular sodium, calcium and magnesium transport [2, 9]. The CaSR enables the ionised calcium level to control renal calcium homeostasis independent of PTH or calcitriol [4].

Claudin-16 and claudin-19 are proteins expressed on the TALH, which facilitate paracellular absorption of divalent cations, including calcium and magnesium [1]. Mutations in claudin-16 are responsible for causing familial hypercalciuria and hypomagnesaemia. Cinacalcet, used for the treatment of secondary hyperparathyroidism in chronic kidney disease, increases claudin-14 mRNA, which subsequently stimulates CaSR activity and decreases paracellular calcium reabsorption [9, 10]. Additionally, PTH and calcitonin upregulate active calcium reabsorption at the TALH [1].

The distal convoluted tubule (DCT) and collecting duct (CD) are responsible for calcium regulation. Around 5–10% of calcium reabsorption occurs through active transport in the DCT, and this mechanism is entirely transcellular [1, 4]. Firstly, calcium travels across the apical membrane by the protein transient receptor potential vanilloid 5 (TRPV5). During this transport process, intracellular calcium is bound to calbindin-D28k and moves towards the basolateral membrane. Finally, calcium reabsorption happens with the help of the sodium-calcium exchanger (NCX1) in conjunction with the plasma membrane calcium ATPase (PMCA1b). This process is represented in **Figure 2** [1, 8].

It is unclear how calcium is transported in the CD; however, a small amount of calcium is thought to be reabsorbed here [2].

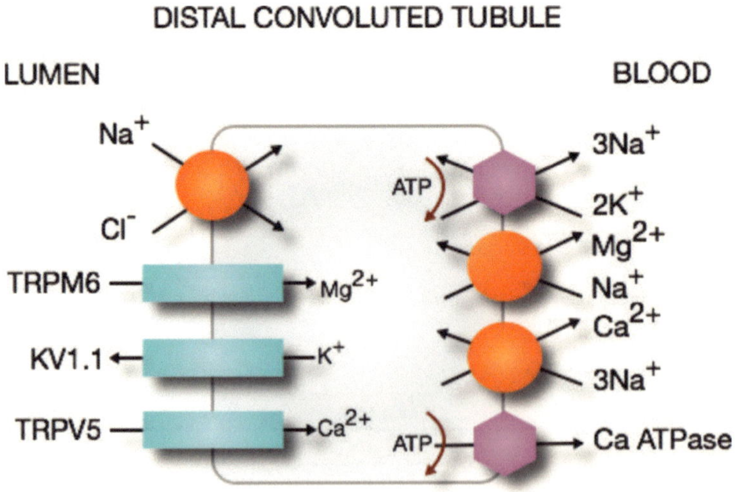

Figure 2. Calcium reabsorption at the distal convoluted tubule. The protein transient receptor potential vanilloid 5 (TRPV5) carries calcium across the apical membrane. Intracellularly calcium binds to calbindin-D28k travelling to the basolateral membrane. The sodium-calcium exchanger (NCX1) and the plasma membrane calcium ATPase reabsorb calcium into the blood [1].

Many mechanisms regulate TRPV5 and therefore renal calcium handling. Mice with absent TRPV5 are known to have hypercalciuria despite normal serum levels of calcium. Their ability to maintain healthy serum calcium levels is believed to be due to increased intestinal absorption mediated by TRPV6 [11]. Calcitriol increases all proteins responsible for transport. Similarly, PTH stimulates TRPV5 and NCX1 while indirectly encouraging calcium reabsorption through the upregulation of calcitriol synthesis. TRPV5, NCX1 and calbindin-D28k are promoted by oestrogen [2].

2.3.2. *Gastrointestinal handling of calcium*

Not all dietary calcium is absorbed as calcium binds with anions (including phosphate and oxalate) in the intestinal lumen to form insoluble salts. Daily intestinal calcium absorption remains relatively constant (200–400 mg per day) despite fluctuations in dietary calcium intake [4, 8].

Gastrointestinal calcium absorption occurs by both transcellular and paracellular mechanisms. The duodenum is the primary site where calcium is absorbed although it also occurs throughout the rest of the small bowel and colon. Transcellular transport is initially mediated by the TRPV6 channel seen on the apical membrane of the duodenum and proximal jejunum [8]. Similar to transcellular absorption in the DCT, once calcium is intracellular, it binds to calbindin, which helps transport the calcium to the basolateral membrane. Here, it is absorbed by calcium ATPase in conjunction with the sodium-calcium exchanger. This is a saturable form of absorption upregulated by calcitriol [2].

In the presence of high luminal calcium concentrations, the passive paracellular pathway of absorption predominates and this is driven by the large concentration gradient between the lumen and cell. This process is nonsaturable. Calcium is bound to the calmodulin-actin-myosin I complex and travels to the basolateral membrane by microvesicular movement [1, 12]. Calcitriol increases calbindin levels and also indirectly influences this process by changing the intracellular tight junction structure [1].

Renal calcium excretion prevents dietary calcium overload, while renal reabsorption and bone resorption compensate for lack of transcellular uptake in the context of low dietary calcium.

2.3.3. *Bone handling of calcium*

Bone acts as a reservoir of calcium stored as hydroxyapatite ($Ca_{10}(PO_4)_6(OH)_2$). Trabecular bone is 15–25% calcified, while cortical bone is 80–90% calcified. Bone acts as an endocrinological organ by offering a readily exchangeable calcium pool, which is used to maintain calcium homeostasis while also allowing bone modelling and remodelling [2].

At any moment, 15–20% of bone is remodelling, facilitated by osteoblasts and osteoclasts. Osteoblasts are formed for pluripotent mesenchymal stem cells. When activated they assist with osteoclastogenesis, bone matrix production and bone mineralisation [13]. Osteoclasts, derived from circulating myeloid cells, are responsible for bone resorption by disrupting bone matrix mineralisation [2, 13].

Many factors influence bone homeostasis. Receptor activator of NF-κB ligand (RANKL) promotes osteoclast production. Osteoprotegerin (OPG) is a soluble receptor, which binds to RANKL and, in doing so, inhibits osteoclast formation. The balance between RANKL and OPG determines the production and function of osteoclasts. PTH activates a PTH receptor (PTH1R) found on osteoblasts. When stimulated, PTH1R upregulates signalling, which favours osteoclast differentiation and bone resorption [13]. The sclerostin/Wnt/beta-catenin pathway also plays a role in controlling bone remodelling whereby sclerostin, which is found in osteocytes, inhibits the Wnt/beta-catenin pathway that works to promote bone formation [2].

2.3.4. Parathyroid hormone and calcium homeostasis

PTH is a polypeptide secreted from stowed granules in the parathyroid gland. Subsequently, metabolisation occurs in the liver and kidney. PTH causes increased plasma calcium levels when hypocalcaemia is detected by CaSRs located on parathyroid cells. It does this by encouraging bone resorption, stimulating intestinal absorption of calcium, upregulating calcitriol production in the kidney (by helping 1-α-hydroxylase that converts vitamin D to calcitriol) and increasing renal calcium reabsorption [1, 2, 4, 8]. PTH is the most significant modulator of calcium reabsorption in the kidney.

PTH secretion is modified by PTH gene transcription, which is upregulated by hypocalcaemia, glucocorticoids and oestrogen. On a post-transcriptional level, PTH is released in reaction to hypocalcaemia, adrenergic agonists, dopamine and prostaglandins [1]. Hypercalcaemia stimulates intracellular destruction of PTH. Calcitriol inhibits PTH gene transcription by binding to the vitamin D receptor element (VDRE) on the PTH gene [2].

2.3.5. Parathyroid hormone-related peptide and calcium homeostasis

The discovery of parathyroid hormone-related peptide (PTHrP) was made when investigating the association between malignancy and hypercalcaemia [14]. Many cells produce PTHrP, which has a similar function and structure to PTH and subsequently activates the same receptor as PTH. It is essential endochondral bone formation, smooth muscle relaxation and cellular proliferation and differentiation; however, it appears to have a limited role in calcium homeostasis in healthy adults [4, 15].

PTHrP is known to be released by both solid organ and haematological malignancies, particularly squamous cell carcinoma. It results in a paraneoplastic hypercalcaemia as it binds to the PTH/PTHrP receptor causing calcium resorption from bone and renal calcium reabsorption. PTHrP-mediated hypercalcaemia is a poor prognostic marker in an individual with a malignancy [16].

2.3.6. Cholecalciferol, calcitriol and calcium homeostasis

The fat-soluble steroid vitamin D3 (cholecalciferol) is found in the diet and synthesised from 7-dehydrocholesterol under the influence of ultraviolet (UV) light. Subsequently, it undergoes hydroxylation by the hepatic enzyme 25-hydroxylase, resulting in 25-hydroxyvitamin D (calcidiol). Calcidiol circulates bound to vitamin D-binding protein where tubular cells that release 1-α-hydroxylase and 24-α-hydroxylase convert calcidiol to 1,25-dihydroxycholecalciferol (calcitriol) and 24,25-dihydroxycholecalciferol. 24,25-Dihydroxycholecalciferol is an inactive metabolite of vitamin D3 [1, 2, 8, 17]. This process is depicted in **Figure 3**.

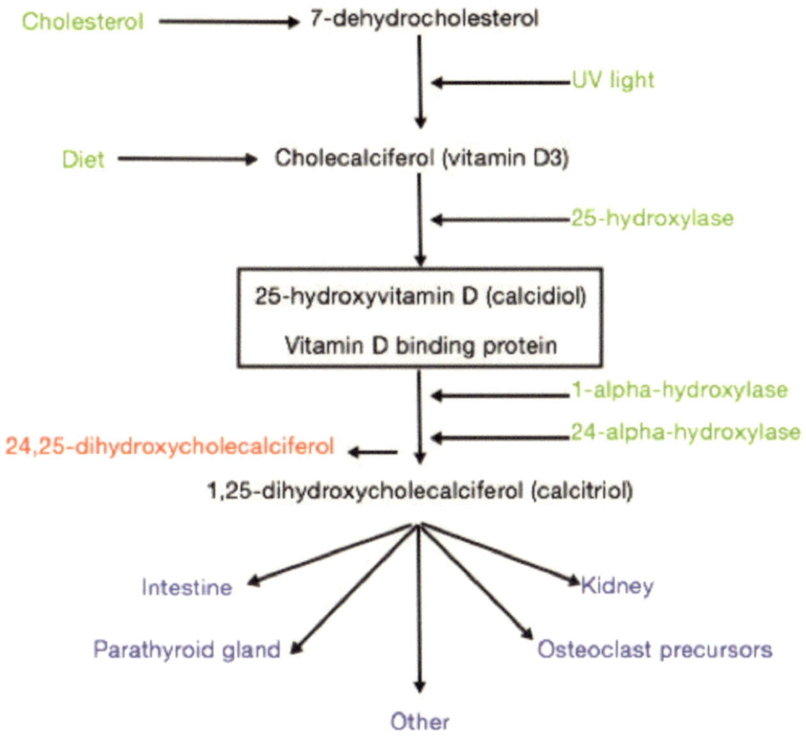

Figure 3. Overview of the metabolism of calcitriol ($1,25(OH)_2D$). Vitamin D_3 (cholecalciferol) is synthesised from 7-dehydrocholesterol in the presence of UV light and is present in the diet (along with vitamin D_2). It is hydroxylated by the hepatic enzyme 25-hydroxylase resulting in 25-hydroxyvitamin D (calcidiol). Calcidiol circulates bound to vitamin D binding protein. Tubular cells release 1-α-hydroxylase (CYP27B1) and 24-α-hydroxylase, which convert calcidiol to 1,25-dihydroxycholecalciferol (calcitriol) and 24,25-dihydroxycholecalciferol.

Calcitriol increases renal reabsorption of calcium and intestinal absorption of calcium and phosphate, increases the mineralisation of bone and reduces PTH synthesis.

2.3.7. Fibroblast growth factor 23, klotho and calcium homeostasis

Fibroblast growth factor 23 (FGF23) is comprised of 251 amino acids and is produced by osteocytes during bone remodelling. Klotho, expressed in the kidney, parathyroid gland, skeletal muscle and choroid plexus, is a coreceptor for FGF23. Klotho upregulates the affinity of FGF23 to its receptors [18]. FGF23 production causes reduction in calcitriol levels as it blocks 1-α-hydroxylase in the kidney causing increased 24-hydroxylase, which, in turn, causes vitamin D degradation. Additionally, it inhibits PTH release. PTH and hypercalcaemia stimulate FGF23, whereas calcitriol and hypocalcaemia impede its production [19].

FGF23 and klotho also play an important role in phosphate homeostasis, which will be discussed later in the chapter.

2.4. Hypercalcaemia

Hypercalcaemia is a result of disrupted calcium homeostasis and can be caused by alterations to organs, hormones or transporters involved in calcium regulation.

Increased intestinal absorption can be secondary to increased calcium intake, as seen in milk-alkali syndrome, or calcium supplementation [20]. Elevated calcitriol can be seen in primary hyperparathyroidism, T cell lymphomas and vitamin D intoxication. Granulomatous diseases (sarcoidosis, tuberculosis) also cause a rise in calcitriol due to autonomous 1-α-hydroxylase activity in macrophages within granulomas. Increased levels of calcitriol stimulate intestinal absorption of calcium as well as renal calcium reabsorption. Hyperparathyroidism, increased PTHrP, bony metastases, myeloma, phosphate depletion, immobilisation and metabolic acidosis lead to increased bone resorption, which may result in hypercalcaemia. Inability to produce bone, as seen in adynamic bone disease, can also lead to hypercalcaemia. Finally, high calcium levels can be a result of decreased renal excretion of calcium due to volume depletion, thiazide diuretic use or alkalosis [3].

Familial hypocalciuric hypercalcaemia is an autosomal dominant condition caused by a mutation, resulting in loss of function in the CaSR gene. It creates hypocalciuria in the setting of hypercalcaemia, associated with hypophosphataemia, hyperchloraemia and hypermagnesaemia. Patients are mostly asymptomatic although severe hyperparathyroidism can occur in affected neonates [21].

2.4.1. Clinical manifestations of hypercalcaemia

Patients with hypercalcaemia can be asymptomatic at time of presentation or can present with any or all of the following: fatigue, mood changes, confusion, nausea, vomiting, loss of appetite, constipation, polyuria, and weakness. Symptoms are seen more often once calcium levels are greater than 2.9 mmol/L (11.6 mg/dL) or in the setting of acute changes to serum calcium levels. Hypercalcaemia can cause cardiac conduction defects including a short QT interval, which may potentiate a cardiac arrhythmia. Renal tubular damage and calcification involving the vasculature, kidneys, skin, lungs, heart and stomach may follow, especially in the setting of normophosphataemia or hyperphosphataemia. Calcium levels above 3.7 mmol/L (14.8 mg/dL) can result in a comatose state or a cardiac arrest. Renal calculi are associated with chronic hypercalcaemia [4, 22].

2.4.2. Treatment of hypercalcaemia

It is essential to consider and treat the underlying aetiology when managing hypercalcaemia. Treatment approaches depend on the severity and symptomatology of the patient. For mild hypercalcaemia (few symptoms or calcium of <3 mmol/L (<12 mg/dL)), treatment with supportive measures while addressing the underlying disease is appropriate. Intravenous fluids can be used to restore euvolaemia in order to reduce PCT calcium reabsorption and enhance calcium excretion. Avoiding calcium-containing medications and maintaining a low calcium diet is necessary for ongoing management [22].

In those with significant symptoms or calcium levels >3 mmol/L (>12 mg/L), more aggressive therapy is warranted. Intravenous fluids remain the first step in treatment, and the rate of administration is mainly governed by the degree of hypercalcaemia. Fluid administration is thought to lower serum calcium levels by 0.5 mmol/L (2 mg/dL). Loop diuretics can be used once the volume state is restored to prevent renal calcium reabsorption. However, with the introduction of bisphosphonate therapy for the management of hypercalcaemia, loop diuretics are less frequently utilised unless the patient is suffering from hypervolaemia, oliguric renal failure or congestive cardiac failure [22].

Calcitonin, produced by parafollicular C cells in the thyroid, is effective in lowering serum calcium quickly in cases of severe hypercalcaemia. It acts by blocking osteoclasts and promoting calciuria. Unlike bisphosphonates and steroids, calcitonin works within 4–6 hours; however its effect only lasts for 48–72 hours, because of rapid development of tachyphylaxis, and therefore, it requires administration in conjunction with a longer-acting treatment strategy [22].

Bisphosphonates (particularly, intravenous pamidronate and zoledronate) are used for malignancy-related hypercalcaemia as they inhibit osteoclast action and, therefore, bone resorption. They take 24–48 hours to work. Dose and infusion rate needs to be adjusted to the patient's renal function [23], and risks of treatment include jaw osteonecrosis, uveitis and nephrotoxicity. Denosumab, an antibody against RANKL, has also been used for the treatment of hypercalcaemia of malignancy and has proven effective in bisphosphonate-resistant disease [24].

In calcitriol-mediated hypercalcaemia (e.g., sarcoidosis, tuberculosis), corticosteroids, in conjunction with a low calcium diet, are adequate. Steroids work by inhibiting 1-α-hydroxylase so that calcidiol is unable to be converted to calcitriol.

In those with a parathyroid adenoma causing primary hyperparathyroidism and resultant hypercalcaemia, surgical removal of the adenoma is necessary.

Due to the availability of bisphosphonates, the need for dialysis in hypercalcaemia has been reduced, but it continues to play a role in individuals with oliguric acute kidney injury, life-threatening manifestations of hypercalcaemia or states refractory to other treatment strategies [4].

2.5. Hypocalcaemia

As previously discussed, PTH is essential in maintaining calcium homeostasis, and in hypoparathyroidism (hereditary or acquired), the absence of PTH means that serum calcium levels are unable to be preserved. Severe hypomagnesaemia (<0.4 mmol/L or <0.8 meq/L) can cause hypocalcaemia as it paradoxically impairs PTH release and causes PTH resistance [4]. Dietary deficiency, anticonvulsant therapy, malabsorption, hepatobiliary disease, renal failure and lack of sunlight cause vitamin D deficiency, leading to hypocalcaemia. Drastic reductions in extracellular calcium levels, seen in pancreatitis, severe acute hyperphosphataemia and rhabdomyolysis, lead to hypocalcaemia as PTH is unable to compensate quickly enough to maintain homeostasis.

2.5.1. Clinical manifestations of hypocalcaemia

The level of calcium and the rate of change will determine the manifestation of symptoms in hypocalcaemia. Common symptoms of hypocalcaemia include fatigue, weakness, irritability, confusion and mood changes. Pathognomonic signs of hypocalcaemia are Trousseau's sign (carpopedal spasm occurs when a blood pressure cuff inflated above the systolic blood pressure) and Chvostek's sign (facial muscle spasm following tapping over the facial nerve) [25]. These signs occur due to neuromuscular excitability [26]. Individuals can also complain of lip paraesthesia, cramping and may experience laryngospasm, bronchospasm, frank tetany or seizures. Cardiac arrhythmias can also occur as low calcium can cause a prolonged QT interval. Chronic hypocalcaemia is associated with cataracts, brittle nails, dry skin and reduced body hair [21].

2.5.2. *Treatment of hypocalcaemia*

Hypocalcaemia is potentially life-threatening, and any individual experiencing laryngospasm, bronchospasm or seizures should be treated immediately with intravenous calcium. Calcium gluconate can be given peripherally as it causes less local irritation than calcium chloride, which requires administration by central venous access [27]. Patients receiving intravenous calcium should be cardiac monitored as rapid correction can also precipitate arrhythmias [26]. Hypomagnesaemia associated with hypocalcaemia requires treatment with intravenous magnesium initially, followed by calcium correction. Less acute presentations of hypocalcaemia can be treated with oral calcium supplementation (e.g., calcitriol). The daily replacement dose can be between 2 and 4 g of elemental calcium.

Treatment of the underlying cause of hypocalcaemia is essential. In cases of hypocalcaemia due to hypoparathyroidism, treatment with calcium leads to increased calciuresis, which may result in nephrocalcinosis and renal impairment. To reduce calciuresis, thiazide diuretics can be used in association with reduced salt and increased fluid intake. Regular monitoring of serum calcium levels is required.

3. Phosphate

3.1. The importance of phosphate

Phosphate plays a role in skeletal integrity, skeletal development, cell structure, cellular signalling, protein synthesis and energy metabolism [28]. Eighty-five percent of biological phosphorus is stored in the bone, while 15% is found in soft tissue. The remaining phosphate (<1%) circulates in the extracellular fluid [29].

Similar to calcium homeostasis, phosphate balance relies on a complex relationship between the intestine, kidneys, bone, as well as regulatory hormones including PTH, FGF23 and klotho.

3.2. Dietary phosphorus

Humans consume between 700 and 2000 mg of dietary phosphorus each day. Phosphorus is present in dairy and protein-rich foods including meat and poultry. It is frequently added to salt and processed foods. With the increase in consumption of processed foods, average dietary intake has increased [30]. In the human body, phosphorus is present in the form of phosphate [1].

3.3. Physiology of phosphate

The majority, 85%, of phosphate in the body exists as bone. The remaining balance of phosphate is present as free anions or forms organophosphate compounds. Organophosphate compounds act as structural proteins, enzymes, transcriptional factors, nucleic acids, energy (adenosine triphosphate, creatine phosphate), carbohydrates and lipids [4].

Normal serum phosphate levels in adults range between 0.75 and 1.45 mmol/L (2.5–4.5 mg/dL). Serum phosphate levels do not always reflect available phosphate levels given that phosphate moves freely between the extracellular and intracellular compartments [4].

3.3.1. Renal handling of phosphate

Regulation of renal phosphate reabsorption is felt to be the most critical mechanism in phosphate homeostasis [8, 29]. Each day, 4–6 g of phosphate is filtered by glomeruli.

Eighty-five percent of phosphate undergoes reabsorption at the PCT. This occurs via the type II sodium-phosphate cotransporters Npt2a (SLC34A1) and Npt2c (SLC34A3) located on the brush border of the apical membrane [28, 31]. These cotransporters are endocytosed, favouring phosphaturia, in the presence of PTH, high dietary phosphorus or FGF23. They have a rapid response to changes in the PTH level, with the number of cotransporters adjusting within minutes. It takes approximately 2 hours for the number of cotransporters to change based on dietary phosphorus intake [28]. Npt2c is thought to have less of an influence on phosphate homeostasis in mice as Npt2a knockout mice continue to have profound phosphaturia despite the presence of Npt2c. However, this cotransporter may play a more significant role in human phosphate homeostasis [28]. In humans, mutations in Npt2c lead to hereditary hypophosphataemic rickets with hypercalciuria (HHRH) compared with mutations in Npt2a, which are characterised by the development of nephrocalcinosis and increased osteoporotic risk. These findings support the importance of the Npt2c cotransporter in human phosphate balance [28, 32, 33].

The type III sodium-phosphate cotransporter, PiT2, has been located in the kidney, also at the brush border membrane. This transporter is upregulated by low dietary phosphate, albeit more slowly than the type II sodium-phosphate cotransporters, with changes in concentrations taking 8 hours [28].

Npt2a and 2c are responsible for transporting divalent phosphate with Npt2a, moving three sodium ions and one phosphate ion across the apical membrane creating an electrogenic gradient. Npt2c transports two sodium and one phosphate ion, resulting in electroneutrality. PiT2 carries monovalent phosphate, also developing an electrogradient [1]. An unknown transporter on the basolateral membrane is thought to be responsible for phosphate transport to peritubular capillaries. This is represented in **Figure 4**.

Hypocalcaemia, hypomagnesaemia, hypophosphataemia and dehydration inhibit reabsorption of phosphate at the kidney. Fluid overload upregulates phosphate excretion [4].

3.3.2. Intestinal handling of phosphate

Different species display diverse mechanisms for intestinal absorption of phosphate, and therefore the understanding of human intestinal phosphate handling is incomplete [34].

Intestinal phosphate absorption occurs via passive paracellular and active transcellular transport. In healthy humans, 60–75% of dietary phosphorus is absorbed [4, 21]. Paracellular transport involves passive diffusion of phosphate through tight junctions and occurs independently

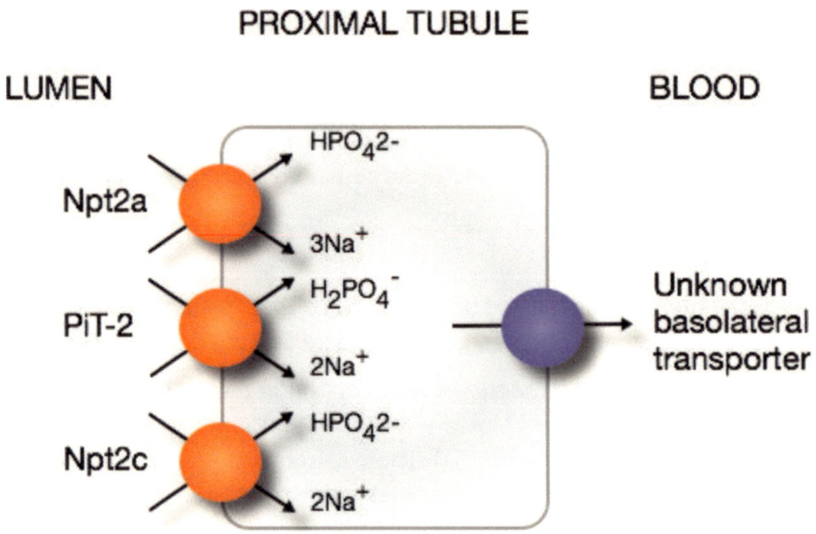

Figure 4. Sodium-phosphate cotransporters at the proximal convoluted tubule. Npt2a, Npt2c and PiT2 are located on the brush border of the apical membrane. Npt2a and 2c transport divalent phosphate. Npt2a transports three sodium ions with one phosphate ion, creating an electrogenic gradient. Npt2c moves two sodium ions for one phosphate, which is electroneutral. PiT2 carries monovalent phosphate creating an electrogradient. An unknown transporter on the basolateral membrane transports phosphate to peritubular capillaries [1].

of any regulatory hormones [34]. The type II sodium-phosphate cotransporter, Npt2b (SLC34A2), and type III cotransporters, PiT1 and PiT2, modulate transcellular transport in the intestine. Npt2b is located on the apical membrane of enterocytes and is thought to be most abundant in the duodenum and jejunum in humans [1] although it is also found on lung, mammary, liver, and testis tissue [31, 34]. Mutations in Npt2b transporters do not manifest in clinically significant hypophosphataemia in humans, and this is thought to be due to renal compensation [28]. The type III cotransporters are predominately present on the basolateral intestinal membrane but can be found on the apical membrane [35].

Gastrointestinal absorption of phosphate is primarily upregulated by calcitriol and low dietary phosphate. FGF23 reduces the abundance and activity of sodium-phosphate cotransporters and will be discussed further in this chapter. Matrix extracellular phosphoglycoprotein (MEPE) produced by osteoblasts and osteocytes inhibits renal and intestinal phosphate absorption independent of PTH and FGF23 [34]. Other regulators of phosphate absorption are glucocorticoids, oestrogen and the presence of metabolic acidosis [28]. Calcium salts, sevelamer hydrochloride and aluminium hydroxide prevent intestinal absorption of phosphate and are therefore used as phosphate binders in patients with chronic kidney disease [4].

3.3.3. Bone handling of phosphate

Similar to calcium, bone acts as a reservoir of phosphate. Phosphate can be resorbed from bone into the extracellular space to maintain serum levels of phosphate.

3.3.4. Fibroblast growth factor 23, klotho and phosphate homeostasis

FGF23 is the most widely studied phosphatonin and acts with its coreceptor, klotho. Dietary phosphorus and calcitriol increase the secretion of FGF23, which encourages phosphaturia through reduced Npt2a expression in the PCT. It plays a similar role in downregulating Npt2c and PiT2; however, in mice studies, this effect has been less pronounced [36]. Conversely, low dietary phosphorus inhibits FGF23 secretion.

FGF23 also contributes to phosphate homeostasis by regulating the number of intestinal sodium-phosphate cotransporters [1]. Similar to the kidney, cotransporters are less abundant in the presence of high levels of FGF23, preventing absorption of phosphorus.

Animal and in vitro studies have proved that FGF23 works directly on the parathyroid gland to decrease PTH production and release [37]. In chronic kidney disease, the parathyroid becomes increasingly resistant to the action of FGF23, contributing to the development of secondary and tertiary hyperparathyroidism [1]. As previously stated, FGF23 also inhibits calcitriol, preventing intestinal phosphate absorption and renal reabsorption [19].

3.3.5. PTH and phosphate homeostasis

PTH reduces the number of sodium-phosphate cotransporters, specifically Npt2a, in the kidney favouring phosphaturia [32, 37]. Serum phosphate levels have a direct effect on the parathyroid gland independent of calcitriol, calcium levels or FGF23. This is mediated by modulation of PTH gene expression and parathyroid cell proliferation [37] but requires intact and functioning parathyroid tissue [38].

3.4. Hyperphosphataemia

Hyperphosphataemia is most often associated with impairment in the kidney's ability to excrete appropriate levels of phosphate [37]. Acute kidney injury leads to hyperphosphataemia due to a reduction in glomerular filtration rate [21]. In early chronic kidney disease, increased phosphate levels are compensated for by FGF23 initially, followed by PTH. With time and a further decrease in glomerular filtration (specifically, at less than an eGFR of 35 $mL/min/1.73^2$), these mechanisms are unable to accommodate due to loss of renal mass meaning that phosphate levels rise. Impaired calcitriol synthesis and bone mineralisation also contribute to elevated phosphate levels. Hyperphosphataemia drives secondary hyperparathyroidism and increased FGF23, which is common in patients with end-stage kidney disease [29]. FGF23 suppresses calcitriol with resultant adverse effects on cardiovascular and kidney health.

Other causes for hyperphosphataemia are driven by elevated exogenous phosphate, as seen following administration of phosphate enemas or excess endogenous phosphate. Bisphosphonate treatment can cause elevated phosphate levels due to the liberation of phosphate from bone. Rapid release of intracellular phosphate into the extracellular space is seen in rhabdomyolysis, tumour lysis syndrome and acidosis [29, 39]. As PTH has a significant influence on promoting phosphaturia, loss of PTH caused by hypoparathyroidism or peripheral resistance to its action (pseudohypoparathyroidism) can produce elevated phosphate levels

[21]. Familial tumoral calcinosis, an autosomal recessive disease caused by a mutation in the GALNT3, FGF23 or klotho gene, is characterised by resistance to FGF23, which also leads to hyperphosphataemia [40]. Increased levels of growth hormone and insulin-like growth factor 1 (Igf-1) seen in acromegaly stimulate phosphate reabsorption in the PCT.

3.4.1. Clinical manifestations of hyperphosphataemia

Acute hyperphosphataemia results in soft tissue calcium and phosphate deposition contributing to hypocalcaemia. These individuals may present with manifestations of hypocalcaemia or with consequences of calcium phosphate deposition including nephrocalcinosis or heart block [4]. Chronic elevation in phosphate levels can lead to vascular calcification, mineral bone disease, secondary hyperparathyroidism and calciphylaxis.

Elevated phosphate levels in patients requiring haemodialysis for end-stage kidney disease is associated with an increased risk of cardiovascular morbidity and mortality [41, 42].

Elevated FGF23 levels, seen in individuals with hyperphosphataemia, have been found to contribute to left ventricular hypertrophy, reduced erythropoiesis and increased inflammation [36].

3.4.2. Treatment of hyperphosphataemia

Acute hyperphosphataemia is managed with intravenous fluids, renal replacement therapy and treatment of the underlying cause [21].

Management of hyperphosphataemia remains a challenge in patients with chronic kidney disease. Low phosphate diets, phosphate binders and dialysis are all used as treatment strategies to maintain healthy phosphate levels. Intensive dialysis (daily or nocturnal dialysis) has been shown to decrease the requirement for phosphate binders and dietary restriction [43].

3.5. Hypophosphataemia

Hypophosphataemia can be caused by impaired phosphate absorption, increased phosphate loss or movement of phosphate from the extracellular space. Reduced phosphate consumption is rare but seen in individuals who are not eating and in those who abuse alcohol. Hypophosphataemia is a known consequence of refeeding syndrome. Primary hyperparathyroidism often presents with mild hypercalcaemia and hypophosphataemia.

Inherited disorders including autosomal dominant, autosomal recessive or X-linked hypophosphataemic rickets and vitamin D-dependent rickets cause excess phosphate loss associated with skeletal deformities. Primary hyperparathyroidism encourages downregulation of NPT2a, resulting in phosphaturia. Proximal tubular dysfunction occurs in proximal tubular acidosis or Fanconi syndrome and contributes to phosphate loss. Hypophosphataemia is common following renal transplantation and is thought to be secondary to persistently elevated FGF23 levels [21].

Causes of intracellular redistribution of phosphate include diabetic ketoacidosis, acute respiratory alkalosis, likely due to muscular sequestration of extracellular phosphate (chronic respiratory alkalosis leads to hyperphosphataemia) and insulin therapy. If phosphate is omitted from TPN, it can cause reductions in serum phosphate. Rarely, mesenchymal tumours such as haemangiopericytomas, fibromas and angiosarcomas can secrete phosphatonins such as FGF23. Subsequently, this results in phosphaturia and hypophosphataemia.

3.5.1. Clinical manifestations of hypophosphataemia

Hypophosphataemia does not cause clinical sequela until levels are less than 0.65 mmol/L (2 mg/dL). Muscle weakness, including diaphragmatic weakness and reduced cardiac contractility, can be a consequence of hypophosphataemia. Other manifestations include osteomalacia, metabolic encephalopathy, haemolysis, leukocyte dysfunction and thrombocytopaenia [4, 21, 42].

3.5.2. Treatment of hypophosphataemia

Dairy intake or oral phosphate supplementation can treat hypophosphataemia, except in cases of nephrocalcinosis or nephrolithiasis due to urinary phosphate wasting. In the case of severe hypophosphataemia, intravenous replacement should be given. In individuals requiring parenteral nutrition, phosphate needs to be added to any nutritional supplement.

4. Magnesium

4.1. The importance of magnesium

The divalent cation magnesium plays an integral role in neuromuscular activity. On an intracellular level, it is the second most abundant cation [21]. It is essential to the activation of adenosine triphosphate (ATP), intracellular signalling, glycolysis, protein formation, cell growth as well as DNA production and transcription [44]. Given its function at the cellular level, it is essential in the role of many human organs including the heart, vasculature, muscle, bone and central and peripheral nervous systems [44].

The normal plasma level of magnesium is 0.7–1.1 mmol/L (1.7–2.6 mg/dL). Similar to calcium and phosphate homeostasis, the kidney, intestine and bone are essential in maintaining its balance.

4.2. Dietary magnesium

The average daily consumption of magnesium from the diet is 140–360 mg. Many foods including fruits, vegetables, cereals, grains, nuts and legumes contain magnesium [45]. Processed, refined and boiled foods are low in magnesium as are dairy products [44, 45].

4.3. Physiology of magnesium

Around 20–28 g of magnesium is present in an average-sized adult with more than half of this being stored in bone [4, 45]. The remaining magnesium is distributed in muscle and soft tissue, and 1% is found in the extracellular compartment [1, 4, 44]. About 30% of magnesium is bound to protein, including albumin, with 10% bound to ATP, nucleic acids, and phospholipids [1]. The remaining 60% exists in the ionised state; it is physiologically active in this form.

Many essential functions in the human body require magnesium; however, it does not appear that hormones have a significant influence on its balance. The kidney, intestine and bone are primarily responsible for maintaining healthy magnesium levels.

4.3.1. Renal handling of magnesium

Under normal physiological conditions, 2000–2400 mg of magnesium is filtered by the kidney each day. Around 10–20% of filtered magnesium undergoes reabsorption by the PCT. This occurs through a predominately paracellular pathway driven by a transepithelial electrochemical gradient caused by sodium reabsorption [46]. In the TALH, 50–70% of magnesium is reabsorbed, also via a paracellular pathway. A lumen-positive transepithelial gradient driven by NKCC2 and ROMK is required. Loop diuretics inhibit the NKCC2 transporter, resulting in magnesium excretion. Claudin-16 and claudin-19 affect the tight junction permeability at the TALH, also altering magnesium reabsorption [46]. The DCT reabsorbs the remaining 10–15% of magnesium. Here, reabsorption occurs through a transcellular pathway mediated by TRPM6, which is present on the apical surface [46, 47]. Epidermal growth factor (EGF) [48] and the sodium-potassium-ATPase transporter increase TRPM6 and therefore the transport of magnesium. The magnesium-sodium exchanger (SLC41A1) on the basolateral membrane facilitates reabsorption into the peritubular capillaries [49].

Renal magnesium reabsorption is thought to be upregulated by PTH but inhibited by hypermagnesaemia and hypercalcaemia [4].

4.3.2. Gastrointestinal handling of magnesium

Intestinal absorption of magnesium depends on dietary intake, but approximately 40% is absorbed. In humans, this predominately takes place in the jejunum and ileum with a small amount being reabsorbed in the colon [44, 50].

Saturable, transcellular magnesium absorption occurs through TRMP6 and TRMP7 channels [1, 44, 47]. Thirty percent of intestinal magnesium absorption occurs through the transcellular mechanism; however, this increases in the instance of low dietary magnesium intake. In cases of high luminal magnesium, the paracellular route predominately drives transport and accounts for 80–90% of intestinal magnesium uptake.

4.3.3. Bone handling of magnesium

Around 50–60% of bodily magnesium is stored in the bone as hydroxyapatite crystals [46]. Half of this is insoluble with the remainder being freely exchangeable with the extracellular fluid. Magnesium has been found to encourage osteoblast differentiation and proliferation, resulting in reduced bone formation in hypomagnesaemic individuals [51].

4.4. Hypermagnesaemia

Exogenous magnesium is found in oral and intravenous magnesium supplementation, rectal enemas, antacids, laxatives and urethral irrigation solutions [45]. Elevated magnesium levels are seen in patients given exogenous magnesium in the context of renal insufficiency but can occur in the presence of normal renal function [21, 45]. The release of intracellular magnesium into the extracellular space is seen in individuals with severe burns, trauma or shock. Associations with hypermagnesaemia include familial hypocalciuric hypercalcaemia, adrenal insufficiency, hypothyroidism and hypothermia.

4.4.1. Clinical manifestations of hypermagnesaemia

Clinical sequelae caused by hypermagnesaemia can occur with levels greater than 2 mmol/L (4.8 mg/dL). Hypermagnesaemia can cause hypotension as a result of vasodilation. Other manifestations include nausea, vomiting, fatigue, neurological impairment and potentially paralysis. Deep tendon reflexes are lost when serum magnesium is greater than 3 mmol/L. Reduced bowel sounds, facial flushing, dilated pupils and heart block are clinical signs, which may manifest [1, 4].

4.4.2. Treatment of hypermagnesaemia

Hypermagnesaemia requires management by ceasing exogenous magnesium administration. Intravenous hydration and intravenous calcium can be used in symptomatic individuals. Calcium is thought to antagonise the effects of magnesium at the neuromuscular junction. Renal replacement therapy is an option in those with chronic kidney disease.

4.5. Hypomagnesaemia

Gastrointestinal causes for hypomagnesaemia include inadequate dietary magnesium intact, gastrointestinal loss through vomiting or diarrhoea, malabsorption, small bowel surgery and alcoholism [46, 52]. Primary familial hypomagnesaemia caused by TRPM6 mutations can result in reduced gastrointestinal absorption and renal loss.

Excessive renal magnesium loss at the PCT is seen with the use of frusemide and in Bartter syndrome; although this is usually mild due to distal compensation. Hypercalcaemia leads to hypomagnesaemia due to competition for transport at the TALH and CaSR activation [52]. Familial hypomagnesaemia with hypercalciuria can occur in mutations of claudin-16 and 19 [53]. At the DCT, thiazide diuretics and Gitelman syndrome cause urinary magnesium loss. EGF upregulates TRPM6, and therefore EGF receptor inhibitors (cetuximab, panitumumab) contribute to hypomagnesaemia. Nephrotoxic medication such as aminoglycosides, amphotericin B, cisplatin, calcineurin inhibitors, pentamidine and cyclosporine can cause hypomagnesaemia [4].

In refeeding syndrome, recovery from diabetic ketoacidosis, pancreatitis, bony metastatic disease and post-parathyroidectomy magnesium can shift from the extracellular to intracellular space.

Chronic proton pump inhibitor use has been associated with hypomagnesaemia, particularly with concomitant diuretic use [52, 54]. The mechanism behind this has been thought to be due to reduced gastrointestinal absorption although causality remains under investigation [54].

4.5.1. Clinical manifestations of hypomagnesaemia

Hypomagnesaemia can result in mood changes, fatigue, muscular spasm, weakness and neuromuscular excitability, which may manifest as hyperreflexia, carpopedal spasm, seizures and tremor [46]. Prolonged QT intervals and ST depression resulting in cardiac arrhythmias can occur. Hypomagnesaemia may potentiate digoxin toxicity. Due to urinary losses, hypocalcaemia and hypokalaemia are often seen with hypomagnesaemia [21].

4.5.2. Treatment of hypomagnesaemia

Hypomagnesaemia requires treatment with oral or intravenous replacement. Oral magnesium supplementation is not well absorbed when used in high doses and can cause diarrhoea. Individuals presenting with symptoms or cardiac manifestations should be treated promptly with intravenous magnesium [45].

5. Conclusion

Calcium, phosphate and magnesium are electrolytes found in the human body, which rely on tight regulatory control in order to support human life and function. The kidney, intestine and bone are essential in maintaining the fine balance. Diseases affecting any of these organs, or the hormones involved in homeostasis, can disrupt the levels of each electrolyte causing symptomatic and potentially life-threatening consequences.

In addition to the kidney, intestine and bone, calcium relies on PTH, PTHrP, phosphate, cholecalciferol, calcitriol, FGF23 and klotho to maintain normal serum levels in the human body. Individuals with hypercalcaemia and hypocalcaemia can present with asymptomatic or symptomatic disease depending on the severity and chronicity. It is important to manage each condition to prevent immediate and long-term complications.

Phosphate and calcium and dependent on each other with disruption to the balance of one having impacts on the other. Phosphate homeostasis is also reliant on PTH, FGF23 and klotho. Hyperphosphataemia is common in patients with chronic kidney disease and has many long-term ramifications, and hypophosphataemia can lead to severe illness and death.

Magnesium does not appear to rely on hormonal control. It plays important roles in neuromuscular activity. Hypermagnesaemia is rare in cases of normal renal function and is most often a result of exogenous ingestion. Hypomagnesaemia may be due to a wide array of causes and disturbs neuromuscular signalling.

Clinicians require a thorough understanding of the intricacies of calcium, phosphate and magnesium homeostasis in order to prevent, diagnose and manage complications of disturbance.

Author details

Vanessa Heron

Address all correspondence to: vanessaheron1@gmail.com

Darling Downs Hospital and Health Service, Toowoomba, Queensland, Australia

References

[1] Blaine J, Chonchol M, Levi M. Renal control of calcium, phosphate, and magnesium homeostasis. Clinical Journal of the American Society of Nephrology. 2015;**10**(7): 1257-1272. DOI: 10.2215/CJN.09750913

[2] Moe S. Calcium homeostasis in health and in kidney disease. Comprehensive Physiology. 2016;**6**:1781-1800. DOI: 10.1002/cphy.c150052

[3] Felsenfeld A, Rodriguez M, Levine B. New insights in regulation of calcium homeostasis. Current Opinion in Nephrology and Hypertension. 2013;**22**:371-376. DOI: 10.1097/MNH.0b013e328362141e

[4] Bringhurst FR, Demay MB, Krane SM, Kronenberg HM. Bone and mineral metabolism in health and disease. In: Harrison's Principles of Internal Medicine. 19th ed. New York: McGraw Hill Education; 2015. pp. 2454-2466

[5] International Osteoporosis Foundation. Calcium [Internet]. 2017. Available from: https://www.iofbonehealth.org/osteoporosis-musculoskeletal-disorders/osteoporosis/prevention/calcium. [Accessed: April 25, 2018]

[6] Castrop H, Schießl IM. Physiology and pathophysiology of the renal Na-K-2Cl cotransporter (NKCC2). American Journal of Physiology. Renal Physiology. 2014;**307**:991-1002. DOI: 10.1152/ajprenal.00432.2014

[7] Welling PA, Ho K. A comprehensive guide to ROMK potassium channel: Form and function in health disease. American Journal of Physiology. Renal Physiology. 2009;**297**(4):849-863. DOI: 10.1152/ajprenal.00181.2009

[8] Hogan J, Goldfarb S. In: Sterns RH, Lam AQ, editors. Regulation of calcium and phosphate balance. Waltham (MA): UpToDate; 2018. Up-to-Date [database on the Internet] [cited 2018-04-21]. Available from: http://www.uptodate.com

[9] Riccardi D, Brown EM. Physiology and pathophysiology of the calcium-sensing receptor in the kidney. American Journal of Physiology. Renal Physiology. 2010;**298**(3):485-499. DOI: 10.1152/ajprenal.00608.2009

[10] Negri AL. Role of claudins in renal calcium handling. Nefrología. 2015;**23**(4):347-352. DOI: 10.1016/j.nefro.2015.06.011

[11] Gkika D, Hsu YJ, van der Kemp AW, et al. Critical role of the epithelial Ca2+ channel TRPV5 in active Ca2+ reabsorption as revealed by TRPV5/calbindin-D28K knockout mice. Journal of the American Society of Nephrology. 2006;**17**:3020. DOI: 10.1681/ASN.2006060676

[12] Sauvanet C, Wayt J, Pelaseyed T, Bretscher A. Structure, regulation, and functional diversity of microvilli on the apical domain of epithelial cells. Annual Review of Cell and Developmental Biology. 2015;**31**:593-621. DOI: 10.1146/annurev-cellbio-100814-125234

[13] Raggatt LJ, Partridge NC. Cellular and molecular mechanisms of bone remodeling. The Journal of Biological Chemistry. 2010;**285**(33):25103-25108. DOI: 10.1074/jbc.R109.041087

[14] Burtis WJ, Wu T, Bunch C, et al. Identification of a novel 17,000-dalton hormone-like adenylate cyclase-stimulating protein from a tumor associated with humoral hypercalcemia of malignancy. The Journal of Biological Chemistry. 1987;**262**(15):7151-7156

[15] Kronenberg HM. PTHrP and skeletal development. Annals of the New York Academy of Sciences. 2006;**1068**:1-13. DOI: 10.1196/annals.1346.002

[16] Donovan PJ, Achong N, Griffin K, Galligan J, Pretorius CJ, McLeod DSA. PTHrP-mediated hypercalcaemia: Causes and survival in 138 patients. The Journal of Clinical Endocrinology and Metabolism. 2015;**100**(5):2024-2029. DOI: 10.1210/jc.2014-4250

[17] White P, Cooke N. The multifunctional properties and characteristics of vitamin D-binding protein. Trends in Endocrinology and Metabolism. 2000;**11**(8):320-327

[18] Izquierdo MC, Perez-Gomez MV, Sanchez-Niño MD, et al. Klotho, phosphate and inflammation/ageing in chronic kidney disease. Nephrology, Dialysis, Transplantation. 2012;**27**:iv6-iv10. DOI: 10.1093/ndt/gfs426

[19] Wolf M. Forging forward with 10 burning questions on FGF23 in kidney disease. Journal of the American Society of Nephrology. 2010;**21**:1427-1435. DOI: 10.1681/ASN.2009121293

[20] Picolos MK, Lavis VR, Orlander PR. Milk-alkali syndrome is a major cause of hypercalcaemia among non-end-stage renal disease (non-ESRD) inpatients. Clinical Endocrinology. 2005;**63**:566-576. DOI: 10.1111/j.1365-2265.2005.02383.x

[21] Kestenbaum B, Drüeke TB. Disorders of calcium, phosphate and magnesium metabolism. In: Johnson RJ, Feehally J, Floege J, editors. Comprehensive Nephrology. 5th ed. Philadelphia: Elsevier; 2015. pp. 124-141

[22] Sternlicht H, Glezerman IG. Hypercalcaemia of malignancy and new treatment options. Therapeutics and Clinical Risk Management. 2015;**11**:1779-1788. DOI: 10.2147/TCRM.S83681

[23] Kyle RA, Yee GC, Somerfield MR, et al. American society of clinical oncology 2007 clinical practice guideline update on the role of bisphosphonates in multiple myeloma. Journal of Clinical Oncology. 2007;**25**(17):2464-2472. DOI: 10.1200/JCO.2007.12.1269

[24] Hu MI, Glezerman IG, Leboulleuz S, et al. Denosumab for treatment of hypercalcaemia of malignancy. The Journal of Clinical Endocrinology and Metabolism. 2014;**99**(9):3144-3152. DOI: 10.1210/jc.2014-1001

[25] Rehman HU, Wunder S. Trousseau sign in hypocalcemia. CMAJ. 2011;**183**(8):498. DOI: 10.1503/cmaj.100613

[26] Cooper MS, Gittoes NJL. Diagnosis and management of hypocalcaemia. BMJ. 2008;**336**: 1298-1302. DOI: 10.1136/bmj.39582.589433.BE

[27] Shoback DM. Hypocalcemia Management [Internet]. 2015. Available from: https://www.ncbi.nlm.nih.gov/books/NBK344077/ [Accessed: April 21, 2018]

[28] Marks J, Debnam ES, Unwin RJ. Phosphate homeostasis and the renal-gastrointestinal axis. American Journal of Physiology. Renal Physiology. 2010;**299**:285-296. DOI: 10.1152/ajprenal.00508.2009

[29] Komaba H, Fukagawa M. Phosphate–A poison for humans? Kidney International. Supplement. 2016;**90**(4):753-763. DOI: 10.1016/j.kint.2016.03.039

[30] Uribarri J, Calvo MS. Dietary phosphorus intake and health. The American Journal of Clinical Nutrition. 2014;**99**(2):247-248. DOI: 10.3945/ajcn.113.080259

[31] Murer H, Forster I, Biber J. The sodium phosphate cotransporter family SLC34. European Journal of Physiology. 2004;**447**:763-767. DOI: 10.1007/s00424-003-1072-5

[32] Prié D, Torres PU, Friedlander G. Latest findings in phosphate homeostasis. Kidney International. Supplement. 2009;**75**:882-889. DOI: 10.1038/ki.2008.643

[33] Lederer E. Renal phosphate transporters. Current Opinion in Nephrology and Hypertension. 2014;**23**:502-206. DOI: 10.1097/MNH.0000000000000053

[34] Aniteli TM, Ramos de Siqueira F, Machado dos Reis L, et al. Effect of variations in dietary Pi intake on intestinal pi transporters (NaPi-IIb, PiT-1 and PiT-2) and phosphate-regulating factors (PTH, FGF-23 and MEPE). Pflügers Archiv. 2018;**470**:623-632. DOI: 10.1007/s00424-018-2111-6

[35] Forster IC, Hernando N, Biber J, Murer H. Phosphate transporters of the SLC20 and SLC34 families. Molecular Aspects of Medicine. 2013;**34**(2-3):386-395. DOI: 10.1016/j.mam.2012.07.007

[36] Courbebiasse M, Lanske B. Biology of fibroblast growth factor 23: From physiology to pathology. Cold Spring Harbor Perspectives in Medicine. 2018;**8**:1-20. DOI: 10.1101/cshperspect.a031260

[37] Slatopolsky E, Brown A, Dusso A. Calcium, phosphorus and vitamin D disorders in uremia. Contributions to Nephrology. 2005;**149**:261-271. DOI: 10.1159/000085687

[38] De Broe ME. Phosphate: Despite advances in research, the benefits to patients remain limited. Kidney International. 2009;**75**:880-881. DOI: 10.1038/ki.2008.692

[39] Wilson FP, Berns JS. Onco-nephrology: Tumor lysis syndrome. Clinical Journal of the American Society of Nephrology. 2012;**7**:1730-1739. DOI: 10.2215/CJN.03150312

[40] Ramnitz MS, Gafni RI, Collins MT. Hyperphosphatemic Familial Tumoral Calcinosis [Internet]. 2018. Available from: https://www.ncbi.nlm.nih.gov/books/NBK476672/ [Accessed: May 04, 2018]

[41] Block GA, Hulbert-Shearon TE, Levin NW, Port FK. Association of serum phosphorus and calcium x phosphate product with mortality risk in chronic haemodialysis patients: A national study. American Journal of Kidney Diseases. 1998;**31**(4):607-617

[42] Wagner CA, Biber J, Murer H. What goes in must come out—The small intestine modulates renal phosphate excretion. Nephrology, Dialysis, Transplantation. 2007;**22**:3411-3412. DOI: 10.1093/ndt/gfm554

[43] Copland M, Komenda P, Weinhandl ED, McCullough PA, Morfin JA. Intensive hemodialysis, mineral and bone disorder, and phosphate binder use. American Journal of Kidney Diseases. 2016;**68**(5):S24-S32. DOI: 10.1053/j.ajkd.2016.05.024

[44] Rios FJ, Montezano AC, Antunes TT, Touyz RM. Magnesium, vascular function and hypertension. In: Collins JF, editor. Molecular, Genetic, and Nutritional Aspects of Major and Trace Minerals. Academic Press; 2016. pp. 353-364. DOI: 10.1016/B978-0-12-802168-2.00029-4

[45] Swaminathan R. Magnesium metabolism and its disorders. Clinical Biochemist Reviews. 2003;**24**:47-66

[46] De Baaij JH, Hoenderop JG, Bindels RJ. Magnesium in man: Implications for health and disease. Physiological Reviews. 2015;**95**:1-46. DOI: 10.1152/physrev.00012.2014

[47] Schlingmann KP, Wldegger S, Konrad M, Chubanov V, Gudermann T. TRPM6 and TRPM7—Gatekeepers of human magnesium metabolism. Biochimica et Biophysica Acta. 2007;**1772**:813-821. DOI: 10.1016/j.bbadis.2007.03.009

[48] Petrelli F, Borgonovo K, Cabiddu M, Ghilardi M, Barni S. Risk of anti-EGFR monoclonal antibody-related hypomagnesaemia: Systematic review and pooled analysis of randomized studies. Expert Opinion on Drug Safety. 2012;**11**:S9-S19. DOI: 10.1517/14740338.2011.606213

[49] Kolisek M, Nestler A, Vormann J, Schweigel-Röntgen M. Human gene SLC41A1 encodes for the Na+/Mg2+ exchanger. American Journal of Physiology. Cell Physiology. 2012;**302**:318-326. DOI: 10.1152/ajpcell.00289.2011

[50] Vormann J. Magnesium: Nutrition and metabolism. Molecular Aspects of Medicine. 2003;**24**:27-37

[51] Liu C, Yeh J, Aloia J. Magnesium directly stimulates osteoblast proliferation. Journal of Bone and Mineral Research. 1988;**3**:104

[52] Agus ZS. Mechanisms and causes of hypomagnesemia. Current Opinion in Nephrology and Hypertension. 2016;**25**(4):301-307. DOI: 10.1097/MNH.0000000000000238

[53] Godron A, Harambat J, Boccio V, et al. Familial hypomagnesemia with hypercalciuria and nephrocalcinosis: Phenotype-genotype correlation and outcome in 32 patients with CLDN16 or CLDN19 mutations. Clinical Journal of the American Society of Nephrology. 2012;**7**:801. DOI: 10.2215/CJN.12841211

[54] William JH, Danziger J. Magnesium deficiency and proton-pump inhibitor use: A clinical review. Journal of Clinical Pharmacology. 2016;**56**(6):660-668. DOI: 10.1002/jcph.672

Chapter 6

Potassium and Its Disorders

Vinay Srinivasa

Additional information is available at the end of the chapter

http://dx.doi.org/10.5772/intechopen.86848

Abstract

Potassium is the major intracellular cation in the human body. Over 98% of the total body potassium is located within the intracellular compartment. In healthy adults, the total intracellular content of potassium is equivalent to 3000–3500 mmol. Approximately 70% of this amount is found in skeletal muscle with lesser amounts in bone, red blood cells, liver and skin. The extracellular compartment contains 1–2% of the total body potassium. This uneven distribution of total body potassium is the result of an electrogenic pump, Na^+, K^+ ATPase. This pump transports three sodium ions extracellularly in exchange of transporting two potassium ions intracellularly. This mechanism creates a ratio that determines the cell membrane potential. Maintenance of this potassium ratio and membrane potential is vital for normal nerve conduction and muscular contraction.

Keywords: hyperkalemia, hypokalemia, acidosis, alkalosis

1. Potassium physiology and homeostasis

The kidney is responsible for maintaining the total body potassium content by matching intake with excretion. Insulin and catecholamines are primarily responsible for the regulation and distribution of potassium between the intracellular and extracellular compartments [21].

Other factors that can alter the distribution of potassium between compartments include acid-base disorders, plasma osmolarity and exercise. The following section describes the effects of these factors in causing transcellular shifts of potassium.

1.1. Transcellular shifts

1.1.1. Insulin and catecholamines

After a meal, postprandial release of insulin shifts dietary potassium from the extracellular compartment into the intracellular compartment. This trans-cellular shift is mediated by insulin binding to cell surface receptors, which stimulates glucose uptake in insulin-responsive tissues via the glucose transporter protein, GLUT 4.

Furthermore, insulin activates the Na^+, K^+ ATPase pump via increased intracellular CAMP production. This increases cellular uptake of potassium, thereby lowering serum potassium. In contrast to insulin, the effect of potassium regulation by catecholamines is dependent on which adrenergic receptor subtype is activated.

Activation of the beta 2 receptor triggers Na^+, K^+ ATPase, which induces cellular potassium uptake causing a fall in serum potassium. Activation of the alpha 1 receptor has the opposite effect, causing inhibition of Na^+, K^+ ATPase preventing cellular uptake and causing elevated serum potassium levels. These effects have important pharmacological implications. Drugs that block beta 2 receptors tend to increase serum potassium. Likewise, drugs that block the alpha 1 receptors can lower serum potassium.

1.1.2. Aldosterone

Aldosterone alters the distribution of potassium between the extracellular and intracellular compartments. The Na^+, K^+ ATPase pump is activated by aldosterone and causes cellular uptake of potassium. In the absence of altered renal potassium excretion, hypokalemia can result.

Aldosterone can also increase potassium excretion via the kidneys and to some degree by the gastrointestinal tract.

Details on the actions of aldosterone in the renal tubule are further explained in Section 1.5.

1.1.3. Hyperglycemia/hyperosmolality

Hyperglycemia and hyperosmolarity cause water movements from the intracellular to the extracellular compartment. This movement is responsible for solvent drag which transports potassium out of the cell. Additionally, cell shrinkage occurs and increases intracellular potassium concentration. There is feedback inhibition of the Na/K ATPase pump which decreases cellular uptake of potassium, thus normalising intracellular potassium. This creates a concentration gradient that allows for potassium exchange between compartments.

1.1.4. Metabolic acidosis

Metabolic acidosis is associated with abnormal serum potassium. Acidosis caused by inorganic anions such as NH_4Cl and HCl can result in hyperkalemia. The mechanism behind this is not understood. Organic acids such as lactic acid generally do not cause potassium shifts between compartments. Hyperkalemia may be seen in lactic acidosis; this is the result of tissue ischemia causing cellular death and release of intracellular potassium into the extracellular fluid.

1.1.5. Exercise

Exercise has multiple effects on potassium. Contraction of skeletal muscle during heavy exercise results in release of potassium. This in turn signals catecholamine release which stimulates alpha 1 adrenergic receptors to cause potassium to shift out of cells. The increase in extracellular potassium further induces arterial vasodilation in normal blood vessels, thereby increasing skeletal blood flow. Catecholamine release during exercise also activates beta 2 adrenoreceptors which increase skeletal muscle uptake of potassium, regulating potassium and minimising exercise-induced hyperkalemia.

1.2. Dietary intake

According to international dietary guidelines, the recommended dietary intake of potassium should be 90–120 mmol/day [3, 20].

Potassium is absorbed through the gastrointestinal tract and is distributed amongst the intracellular and extracellular fluid compartments. Dietary intake varies worldwide; the western diet provides 50–100 mmol of potassium daily [3, 21].

Foods that are rich in potassium include many fruits and vegetables.

After a potassium-rich meal, increases in extracellular potassium are negated by rapid cellular uptake that allows for elimination in the urine over a period of 6–8 h.

About 90% of potassium is excreted in the urine with the remaining 10% excreted via the stool.

Potassium homeostasis is controlled by the changes in renal potassium excretion. The following section describes the basic physiology of renal potassium excretion.

1.3. Renal potassium excretion

Evolving concepts in renal potassium excretion involves the recognition of reactive and predictive systems [16].

The reactive system comprises of a negative and a forward system. The negative system consists of a negative feedback loop that modulates renal potassium, on the basis of plasma potassium and serum aldosterone levels [16].

High plasma potassium concentrations or elevated serum aldosterone levels increase urinary potassium excretion bringing plasma potassium concentration back to physiologic range. The forward system describes an unidentified potassium-sensing gut factor that increases urinary potassium excretion, in response to a high potassium diet before an increase in plasma potassium concentration, or changes in plasma aldosterone levels occur [4, 5, 7]. In addition to these systems, a circadian rhythm of potassium excretion has been proposed, for instance, the predictive system which is independent of potassium intake and activity. In studies measuring urinary potassium excretion, it has been observed that urinary potassium excretion is the lowest in the night and early mornings and highest from noon to early afternoon [16].

1.4. Renal potassium handling

Serum potassium is almost completely ionised and not bound to plasma proteins. It is filtered through the glomerulus. Approximately 65–70% of potassium filtered through glomeruli is reabsorbed in the proximal tubule. Less than 10% of the filtered load reaches the distal nephron.

Potassium reabsorption in the proximal tubule primarily occurs through paracellular pathways.

Sodium reabsorption across the tubule allows for fluid absorption to occur. As a result of this process, solvent drag occurs which permits potassium reabsorption. In addition, the electrical voltage within the tubular lumen gradually becomes more positive as fluid flows down the tubule.

This change in voltage provides an additional force favouring potassium reabsorption through the paracellular pathway, which is of low resistance.

In the loop of Henle, both secretion and absorption occur. Potassium is secreted in the descending loop in deep nephrons and is reabsorbed in the ascending loop through the action of the Na^+, K^+ $2Cl^-$ cotransporter. The majority of the potassium reabsorbed by this protein is recycled back into the tubular lumen by the renal outer medullary potassium channel (ROMK), an ATP-dependent apical potassium channel that transports potassium out of cells. Modest net absorption of potassium occurs as a result of this process. The site and regulation of renal potassium excretion predominantly occurs in the distal tubule and collecting duct.

The distal nephron, which comprises the distal tubule and collecting duct, has both reabsorptive and secretory functions. Potassium excretion primarily occurs here.

There are several cell types within the epithelium of the distal tubule and collecting ducts. The most important of these cell types are the principal cells, which approximate to 70% of cells and the intercalated cells. Both cell types are located within the collecting duct. Principal cells are primarily located within the cortical collecting duct and intercalated cells are dispersed throughout the entire length of the collecting duct.

Potassium secretion is by principal cells, which involves uptake of potassium from the interstitium by Na^+, K^+ ATPase and secretion into the tubular lumen through potassium channels: ROMK and BK also known as maxi-K.

ROMK and BK are both permeable to potassium and are regulated by different mechanisms [3].

There are several factors that influence principal cells to secrete potassium. These factors include low potassium diet, high potassium diet, angiotensin II, high serum potassium, aldosterone, luminal flow rate, extracellular pH and high Na delivery.

Sodium delivery to the distal tubule is the major regulator of potassium excretion. High sodium delivery stimulates potassium secretion. It achieves this in two ways. Firstly, increased sodium delivery causes increased sodium entry via epithelial sodium channels (ENaC), which depolarises the apical membrane causing an increase in the electrochemical gradient, promoting outward flow potassium through the potassium channels. Secondly, the more sodium delivered to the tubule, the more sodium is pumped out by Na^+, K^+ ATPase and more potassium is pumped in [3].

http://dx.doi.org/10.5772/intechopen.86848

This potassium is then secreted across the apical membrane of principal cells into the luminal fluid by apical potassium channels.

At low dietary loads of potassium, there is no secretion by either channel. The body is conserving potassium. ROMK channels are sequestered into intracellular vesicles. BK channels are closed [3]. In normal concentrations of potassium, ROMK channels secrete potassium whereas BK channels remain closed. In conditions where there is high potassium secretion, for example, high potassium diet, both ROMK and BK channels are open [3].

Angiotensin II is an inhibitor of potassium secretion; its mode of action is to decrease activity of ROMK, thereby limiting potassium flux into the tubular lumen.

The intercalated cells are subdivided into type A which are numerous, type B which are limited in number and non-A and non-B cells.

The intercalated cells, particularly type A, reabsorb potassium. Type A intercalated cells reabsorb potassium via the H^+, K^+ ATPase, located within the apical membrane which actively takes up potassium from the lumen in exchange for hydrogen ions. Potassium can then enter the tubular interstitium across the basolateral membrane via potassium channels. In conditions of low potassium, potassium depletion increases H^+, K^+ ATpase expression resulting in increased active potassium reabsorption and decreased potassium excretion.

An important regulator of potassium in the distal nephron is the enzyme with no lysine kinases (WNK kinases). WNK kinases activate sodium reabsorption in the distal tubule and inhibit the ROMK channel [16, 22].

As a result of this, there is decreased sodium delivery to the collecting duct, and coupled with this is decreased ROMK expression leading to decreased potassium secretion [16, 22].

WNK kinase activity is sensitive to chloride and potassium concentrations [16, 22].

1.5. Aldosterone paradox

Aldosterone has the ability to signal the kidney to cause sodium retention without potassium secretion in states of volume depletion but can also stimulate potassium secretion without sodium retention in the hyperkalemic state [6].

In humans, aldosterone is the major mineralocorticoid. It promotes sodium absorption and potassium excretion by binding to mineralocorticoid receptors located in the distal tubules and collecting ducts. Aldosterone increases Na^+, K^+ ATPase activity in the basolateral membrane which is responsible for sodium reabsorption across the luminal membrane. This increases the electronegativity of the lumen which increases the electrical gradient and potassium permeability.

In states of volume depletion, the renin-angiotensin-aldosterone axis is activated and causes renal sodium absorption restoring extracellular fluid volume without a demonstrable effect on renal potassium excretion. In the presence of hyperkalemia, release of aldosterone increases urinary potassium excretion, thereby restoring serum potassium levels to normal. This effect, however, does not result in sodium renal retention.

2. Disorders of potassium

2.1. Hypokalemia

2.1.1. Epidemiology

Hypokalemia is defined as serum potassium concentration levels of <3.5 mmol and is a common electrolyte disturbance amongst hospitalised patients [6].

As many as 20% of hospitalised patients are found to have hypokalemia, but only 4–5% of this is deemed to be clinically significant [6, 13, 22].

There are no significant differences in its prevalence amongst males and females [6].

2.1.2. Aetiology

2.1.2.1. Redistribution

About 2% of the total body potassium is within the extracellular compartment. Consequently, small shifts of potassium from the extracellular compartment to the intracellular compartment can cause hypokalemia. Additionally, glycogenesis during total parenteral nutrition or enteral hyperalimentation causes insulin release which shifts potassium into cells. Furthermore, the sympathetic nervous system is involved in the activation of the beta 2 receptors causing intracellular shift of potassium. Stimulation of beta 2 receptors can also occur in thyrotoxicosis.

A rare cause of redistribution-induced hypokalemia is hypokalemic periodic paralysis. In this condition, flaccid paralysis and muscular weakness occur during the night or early mornings, typically after ingestion of a large carbohydrate meal.

2.1.2.2. Renal potassium losses

Renal potassium losses are the most common cause of hypokalemia.

Drugs are common causes of renal potassium loss.

Thiazide and loop diuretics block sodium reabsorption in the distal convoluted tubule and loop of Henle, respectively. Reabsorption does not occur proximal to the collecting duct, thereby increasing sodium delivery to the principal cells of the collecting duct. This stimulates sodium uptake and at the same time promotes potassium secretion causing potassium loss resulting in hypokalemia.

High dosage of penicillins is thought to cause hypokalemia by increased sodium delivery to the collecting duct and principal cells which result in urinary potassium secretion [22].

The antifungal agent amphotericin directly increases collecting duct secretion of potassium. This is achieved by its direct action of binding to collecting duct cells and forming pores which result in potassium loss.

http://dx.doi.org/10.5772/intechopen.86848

The mechanism of action for aminoglycosides causing hypokalemia is not completely understood [22]. It is postulated that ROMK is activated by aminoglycosides causing urinary potassium secretion [22].

Cisplatin, an antineoplastic agent can cause both hypokalemia and hypomagnesemia.

Hypokalemia is related to hypomagnesemia. Magnesium mediates inhibition of ROMK. In states that where there is magnesium deficiency, ROMK inhibition is lost enabling potassium excretion [22].

Coupled with this is inhibition of Na^+, K^+ ATPase pump caused by low magnesium, causing potassium to be excreted via K channels particularly in the thick ascending limb [22].

Toluene is thought to lead to potassium wasting by causing renal tubular acidosis (RTA) [22].

Licorice and herbal cough mixtures contain glycyrrhizic and glycyrrhetinic acids. They are thought to exert mineralocorticoid effects leading to hypokalemia [22].

Bicarbonaturia results from metabolic alkalosis, distal RTA or treatment with proximal RTA.

Increased distal tubular bicarbonate delivery increases potassium secretion.

Magnesium deficiency can cause high potassium excretion and potassium deficiency. Under ideal conditions, intracellular magnesium inhibits the apical ROMK channel. In magnesium deficiency, the ROMK channel is not inhibited by magnesium resulting in increased potassium excretion.

Magnesium deficiency should be suspected when potassium replacement does not correct the hypokalemia.

Intrinsic renal potassium transport defects are rare. Barterrs, Gittlemanns and Liddles are such conditions. A review of these conditions is not described here.

Similarly, detailed descriptions of genetic defects that result in elevated levels of aldosterone, glucocorticoid remediable aldosteronism, congenital adrenal hyperplasia and syndrome of apparent mineralocorticoid excess, are not described in great detail here (See **Table 1**).

Drugs	Hormones	Renal tubular defects	Genetic defects
• Thiazide diuretics • Loop diuretics • Penicillins; Piperacillin-Tazobactam • Amphotericin B • Aminoglycosides • Cisplatin • Toluenes • Herbal cough mixtures	• Aldosterone	• Bartter syndrome • Gitelman syndrome • Liddle syndrome	• Glucocorticoid-remediable aldosteronism • Syndrome of apparent mineralocorticoid excess • Congenital adrenal hyperplasia

Table 1. Causes of renal potassium losses.

2.1.2.3. Extra-renal potassium losses

The skin and gastrointestinal tract excrete small amounts of potassium. Excessive sweating or chronic diarrhoea can cause potassium losses. Likewise, vomiting or nasogastric suction can cause hypokalemia although gastric fluids contain only 5–8 mmol/l of potassium. This is associated with concomitant metabolic alkalosis and intravascular volume depletion which cause secondary hyperaldosteronism and increases urinary potassium loss.

2.1.2.4. Pseudohypokalemia

Pseudohypokalemia occurs when serum potassium decreases artifactually after phlebotomy.

Acute leukemia is the most common cause. Abnormal leucocytes take up potassium when blood is stored in collection vial for a prolonged period of time at room temperature. Rapid separation of plasma and storage at 4°C are used for diagnosis.

Clinical features: the clinical manifestations of hypokalemia are proportionate to the degree and duration of serum potassium reduction.

Symptoms are often not present until serum potassium is below 3.0 mmol/L.

A potentiating factor such as digoxin can predispose hypokalemic patients to have cardiac arrhythmias because of altered resting membrane potential.

2.1.2.5. Cardiac

Epidemiological studies have linked hypokalemia and low potassium diet with an increased prevalence of hypertension.

Potassium deficiency can increase blood pressure. Mechanisms that have been proposed to be responsible for this effect include sodium retention with subsequent increased intravascular volume and endogenous vasoconstriction which sensitises the vasculature.

Electrocardiographic (ECG) changes with cardiac arrhythmias can be seen. Common ECG changes are U waves and ST segment depression along with T wave flattening.

2.1.2.6. Hormonal

Hypokalemia impairs insulin release and induces insulin resistance which worsens glycemic control in diabetic patients.

2.1.2.7. Muscular

Hypokalemia can lead to skeletal muscle weakness and increases sensitivity to develop exertional rhabdomyolysis by reducing skeletal muscle blood flow. Furthermore, hypokalemia hyperpolarises skeletal muscle reducing muscle contraction.

2.1.2.8. Renal

Hypokalemia can lead to significant disturbances in renal function.

Reduced medullary blood flow and increased renal vascular resistance may result in hypertension, tubulointerstitial and cystic changes, acid base disturbances and damage to the renal concentrating mechanisms [22].

Potassium deficiency can cause tubulointerstitial fibrosis which is seen in the outer medulla. The duration of hypokalemia determines the degree of damage. Prolonged hypokalemia may result in renal failure. Furthermore, chronic potassium deficiency causes renal hypertrophy that can lead to renal cyst formation particularly during increased mineralocorticoid use [22].

Hypokalemia increases renal ammonia production.

Metabolic alkalosis is associated with hypokalemia and occurs because of increased renal net acid secretion as a result of increased ammonia excretion [22].

Additionally, it can also cause increased urinary potassium secretion resulting in hypokalemia.

In cases of severe hypokalemia, respiratory muscle weakness may arise leading to the development of respiratory acidosis and if severe, respiratory acidosis.

Severe potassium depletion can cause polyuria, with urinary outputs measuring 2–3 L.

Increased thirst and nephrogenic diabetes insipidus are factors potentiating the severity of polyuria. Nephrogenic diabetes insipidus is a result of decreased expression of water transporter aquaporin 2 (AQP2) and urea transporter proteins UT-A1, UT-A3, and UT-B which take part in urine concentration mechanisms and water reabsorption [22].

2.1.2.9. Nervous system

Cramps, paresthesias, paresis, and ascending paralysis are typical features of neurological involvement.

2.1.2.10. Treatment

Treatment approach is dependent on the severity of hypokalemia and the presence of symptoms. Treatment should include reducing the amount of potassium lost, replenishing potassium stores, assessing for potential toxicities, and determining the cause so that future episodes can be prevented [6, 22].

Short-term risks of hypokalemia are cardiovascular arrhythmias and neuromuscular weakness which can be life-threatening and require urgent treatment in the form of intravenous potassium usually 5–10 mmol over 15–20 min [22].

Urgent treatment for hypokalemia however is rarely required [14].

It should be noted that the body responds to potassium losses, by shifting potassium from the ICF compartment to the ECF compartment, minimising change in extra-cellular potassium. With potassium replacement, potassium is shifted back into the ICF. The degree or magnitude of potassium deficiency can be masked. The amount of potassium required to replace the potassium lost is greater than predicted change in extra-cellular volume [6, 22].

The severity of hypokalemia determines the administration of either intravenous or oral potassium. Patients presenting with potassium levels of 2.5–3.5 mmol represent mild to moderate hypokalemia and can be treated with oral potassium supplements. Severe hypokalemia defined as potassium levels of <2.5 mmol should be treated with intravenous potassium [6, 22].

Hypokalemia is associated with magnesium deficiency. Magnesium is important for potassium uptake and for maintenance of intracellular potassium levels particularly in the myocardium [1].

2.1.2.11. Intravenous potassium

Intravenous potassium infusions can cause pain if given peripherally via a small vein. The maximum rate of potassium administration peripherally is 10 mmol/h [1, 6, 22].

In cases where more rapid replacement is necessary, potassium infusion rates >10 mmol/h can be administered but require central access, electrocardiograph monitoring and frequent monitoring of serum potassium [1, 6, 22].

2.1.2.12. Oral potassium

Oral potassium supplements can take the form of potassium chloride or effervescent tablets.

Potassium chloride tablets contain 8 mmol of potassium per tablet, as opposed to effervescent tablets which contain 14 mmol per tablet (**Table 2**).

2.2. Hyperkalemia

2.2.1. Epidemiology

Hyperkalemia occurs frequently amongst patients with chronic kidney disease, diabetes and heart failure and patients using RAAS inhibitors (renin-angiotensin-aldosterone) or NSAIDS (non-steroidal anti-inflammatories). Less than 1% of normal healthy adults develop hyperkalemia [22].

2.2.2. Aetiology

Hyperkalemia can be the result of psuedohyperkalemia, potassium redistribution from intracellular fluid to extracellular fluid and imbalances between potassium intake and excretion.

Hypokalemia	Treatment
Mild (3.0–4.0 mmol)	Oral potassium: • Effervescent tablets1–2 tabs bd (14–28 mmol) • Potassium chloride tablets 1–2 tabs bd (8–16 mmol) • IV potassium; 60 mmol/24 h
Moderate (2.5–3.0 mmol)	Oral requirements; total requirements are 96 mmol/day [2]. IV potassium infusion; 90 mmol/24 h [2]
Severe (<2.5 mmol)	IV potassium infusion: 5–10 mmol/h

Table 2. Treatment of hypokalemia.

In this section, a brief description of each cause is given.

2.2.3. *Psuedohyperkalemia*

Release of potassium from erythrocytes after phlebotomy occurs. Free hemoglobin is released into plasma from damaged erythrocytes and is reported as hemolysis. In the presence of hemolysis, reported plasma potassium is not representative of the actual plasma potassium. Treatment should not be initiated, and repeat measurement of plasma potassium must take place.

Ischemia from difficult phlebotomy or exercise of limb in the presence of tourniquet can lead to abnormally increased potassium values. Potassium can also be released from other cellular elements present in blood during clotting particularly, with severe leucocytosis (>70,000/cm^3) or thrombocytosis. About one-third of patients with platelet counts of 500–1000 × 10^{-9} have psuedohyperkalemia [22].

Diagnosis of psuedohyperkalemia is made by measuring serum/plasma potassium.

2.2.3.1. *Redistribution*

Hyperglycemia from insulin deficiency and hyperosmolarity are important causes of potassium movement from the intracellular fluid to the extracellular fluid. Moreover, medications such as beta 2 adrenoreceptor antagonists, RAAS inhibitors and mineralocorticoid receptor blockers are common agents that can cause hyperkalemia.

2.2.3.2. *Potassium intake*

In general, excessive dietary intake does not cause chronic hyperkalemia because the kidney can excrete ingested potassium.

There are other factors that contribute to hyperkalemia when renal potassium excretion is impaired.

2.2.3.3. *Impaired potassium excretion*

In patients with decreased kidney function, there is impaired potassium excretion.

In chronic kidney disease, renal potassium secretion from distal nephrons is preserved until the glomerular filtration rate is reduced to 10–20 ml/min [22].

Medications can affect potassium excretion. A list of medications and their effects is described in **Table 3**.

Hyperkalemia may occur in obstructive uropathy. This is in part due to decreased Na^+, K^+ ATpase expression and activity. It can persist for months or years after the obstruction is relieved [22].

This is thought to be due to a persistent defect in the collecting duct, where secretion is impaired.

Aldosterone deficiency is not responsible.

Class	Class example	Mechanism
Potassium-containing drugs	Potassium chloride	Increased potassium intake
Beta adrenergic blockers	Propranolol, metoprolol, and atenolol	Inhibition of renin release
Angiotensin-converting enzyme (ACE) inhibitors	Ramipril, perindopril, and lisinopril	Inhibition of angiotensin I to angiotensin II
Angiotensin receptor blockers	Irbesartan, losartan, and candesartan	Inhibition of angiotensin I receptor by angiotensin II
Direct renin inhibitors	Aliskiren	Inhibition of renin activity resulting in decreased angiotensin II production
Heparin	Heparin sodium	Inhibition of aldosterone synthase, rate-limiting enzyme for aldosterone synthesis
Aldosterone receptor antagonists	Spironolactone and eplerenone	Block aldosterone receptor activation
Potassium-sparing diuretics	Amiloride and triamterene	Block collecting duct apical ENaC channel, decreasing gradient for K secretion.
NSAIDS and COX-2 inhibitors	Ibuprofen	Inhibition of prostaglandin stimulation of collecting duct potassium secretion. Inhibition of renin release
Digitalis glycosides	Inhibition of Na^+, K^+ ATPase necessary for collecting duct K secretion and regulation of K distribution into cells.	Digoxin
Calcineurin inhibitors	Inhibition of Na^+, K^+ ATPase necessary for collecting duct K secretion.	Cyclosporine and tacrolimus

Table 3. Pharmacological agents causing hyperkalemia. Class Example and Action description for digoxin and CNI need to be reversed, for eg action of drug for digoxin under class example and class example digoxin is under action of drug, this also applies FOR CNI.

http://dx.doi.org/10.5772/intechopen.86848

2.3. Clinical manifestations

Hyperkalemia may be asymptomatic or cause life threatening arrhythmias.

2.3.1. *Cardiac*

Hyperkalemia decreases the transmembrane potassium gradient. This results in cell membrane depolarisation, slowing of ventricular conduction and decrease in the duration of the action potential. These changes result in electrocardiogram (ECG) manifestations including peaked T waves, broadening of QRS complexes, loss of p wave and ventricular fibrillation which can lead to asystole. Changes in plasma potassium may not result in ECG changes. ECG has been described to be a poor tool for detecting hyperkalemia with a sensitivity of 34–40% [9–12, 15].

2.3.2. *Neuromuscular*

Neuromuscular effects include paresthesias, weakness and paralysis. Deep tendon reflexes may be depressed or absent. Sensory findings are absent.

2.3.3. *Gastrointestinal*

Nausea, vomiting and diarrhoea can occur but are less encountered.

2.4. Diagnosis

Transtubular potassium gradient (TTKG) can help distinguish renal causes of hyperkalemia from non-renal causes.

It is a measurement of net potassium secretion by the collecting duct after correcting for changes in urinary osmolality.

The formula is as follows Eq. (1):

$$\mathrm{TTKG} = \frac{\text{urine potassium} \cdot \text{urine osmolality}}{\text{plasma potassium} \cdot \text{plasma osmolality}} \tag{1}$$

2.4.1. *Effects on the cardiac system*

Calcium given by the parenteral route does not produce changes in extracellular potassium but stabilises cell membrane potential by ameliorating the effects of hyperkalemia on myocardial conduction system and depolarisation [22] (**Tables 4** and **5**).

Responses occur within a few minutes and duration of action is between 30 and 60 min.

Although there are no clinical studies assessing efficacy, it has been accepted for the treatment of hyperkalemia when life threatening ECG changes are present or when cardiac arrest occurs. Life-threatening ECG changes include absent P waves, broad QRS complexes and sine-wave pattern.

TTKG	Indication
<5–7	Suggest aldosterone deficiency or resistance
6–12	Normal
>10	Suggest normal aldosterone action and extra renal cause of increased potassium.

Table from Comprehensive Clinical Nephrology 6th Edition. 2019.

Table 4. Interpretation of TTKG.

Medication	Dose	Route of administration	Time of onset	Mechanism
Calcium gluconate Calcium chloride	Calcium gluconate 10% Calcium chloride 10 mls	Intravenous	1–3 min	Cell membrane stabilisation
Insulin with dextrose	10 units IV with 50 mls of 50% dextrose	Intravenous	30 min	Cellular potassium uptake
Beta 2 adrenergic agonist	Salbutamol 15–20 mg	Nebuliser	30 min	Cellular potassium uptake
Sodium polystyrene sulfonate	30 g–60 g	Oral	>2 h	Potassium removal by potassium binding resins
*Sodium bicarbonate++	25–100 mls 8.4% $NaHCO_3$ over 5–15 minutes	Intravenous	within 60 min	Transcellular shift by alkalinisation Bicarbonate affecting H/K exchange; pushes potassium back into cells.

*Sodium bicarbonate can be considered if acidemia is present; pH <7.2.

++Hemodialysis is the most effective method of removal of potassium. Acute hemodialysis is indicated when hyperkalemia is life threatening and is refractory to medical treatment. The more severe the hyperkalemia is, the more rapid reduction of plasma potassium is required, until serum potassium is <6.0 mmol/L.

Table 5. Treatment of hyperkalemia.

The dose of calcium gluconate is higher than calcium chloride because it requires liver metabolism to release calcium.

2.4.2. Cellular uptake of potassium

Insulin and beta 2 adrenergic agonists stimulate cellular uptake of potassium. Insulin achieves this by binding to insulin receptors located on skeletal muscle. The duration of action for insulin can last for 4–6 h. Glucose is co-administered to prevent hypoglycemia.

Beta 2 receptor adrenergic agonists can be administered via inhalation and subcutaneous or intravenous routes. Tachycardia is a significant complication of therapy particularly at high doses required to treat hyperkalemia (2–8 times higher given for bronchodilation).

It has been reported that upto 25% of patients with hyperkalemia do not respond to beta 2 agonist therapy [17, 19].

2.4.3. *Potassium removal*

Reducing total body potassium involves decreased oral intake, enhanced fecal and urinary potassium excretion and dialysis.

In terms of dietary intake, limited amounts of citrus fruits, potatoes, tomatoes and salt products should be ingested.

Hemodialysis is the most effective mode of removal of potassium. In patients with advanced renal failure, the ability of the distal nephron to excrete potassium is reduced. In these patients, hemodialysis is the preferred mode of removal.

Oral potassium binding resins are other agents used in the treatment of hyperkalemia.

This is best observed in patients with chronic hyperkalemia. Sodium polystyrene sulfonate and calcium polystyrene sulfonate are common agents used. They exchange sodium and calcium, respectively, for potassium in the gastrointestinal tract. It can be administered orally or rectally as a retention enema. Furthermore, polystyrene sulfonates have been reported to cause constipation, intestinal necrosis and colonic perforation. Consequently, newer agents have been developed and are being evaluated in clinic trials.

Sodium zirconium cyclosilicate (ZS-9) is an oral cation exchanger designed to trap monovalent cations in the gastrointestinal tract. Its framework structure is full of micropores that allow selectivity of trapping potassium ions in exchange for sodium and hydrogen. Clinical trials have demonstrated its success in lowering plasma potassium levels within 24 h. The onset of action is 1 h following the first dose. Dose has varied from 2.5 to 10 g. Dose-dependent oedema is a notable side effect. It should be given 2 h apart from oral medications with gastric pH dependence. It binds potassium throughout the gastrointestinal tract. The bioavailability is 7 h after the onset of action after the first dose. Location of potassium binding is predominantly in the distal colon.

Long-term effects on mortality are still yet to be confirmed. In May 2018, the FDA approved ZS-9 for the treatment of hyperkalemia. It is known as Lokelma in the USA.

Patiromer is another new agent that binds potassium in the lumen of the gastrointestinal tract.

It consists of a polymer anion (the active moiety patiromer) and a calcium-sorbitol complex.

Clinical trials have shown a reduction in plasma potassium levels but there are some side effects that have been observed. Hypomagnesemia has been reported in patients taking this agent.

Its use in patients with cardiac arrhythmia has been questioned, as hypomagnesemia can be associated with cardiac arrhythmias. It can also cause gastrointestinal side effects, for example, mild to moderate constipation. Its brand name is Veltessa.

Author details

Vinay Srinivasa

Address all correspondence to: vinay.srinivasa@health.qld.gov.au

Nephrology Advanced trainee, Toowoomba Hospital, Queensland, Australia

References

[1] Alfonzo A, Isles C, et al. Potassium disorders: Clinical spectrum and emergency management. Resuscitation. 2006;**70**:10-25

[2] Ballarat Health Services. Drug Guideline, Potassium—Intravenous infusion and enteral (critical care areas). 2013

[3] Eaton D, Pooler J. Vanders Renal Physiology. 8th ed. New York, USA: Mcgraw Hill Education; 2013

[4] Ellison DH, Terker AS, et al. Potassium and its discontents: New insight, new treatments. Journal of the American Society of Nephrology. 2016;**27**:981-989

[5] Jain G, Ong S, et al. Genetic disorders of potassium homeostasis. Seminars in Nephrology. 2013;**33**(3):265-276

[6] Kardalas E, Paschou S, et al. Hypokalemia: A clinical update. Endocrine Connections. 2018;**7**:135-146

[7] Kollef MH, Bedient TJ ea. Washington Manual of Critical care. USA: Lipincott Williams and Wilkins; 2008

[8] Kovesdy CP, Matsushita K, Sang Y, et al. Serum potassium and adverse outcomes across the range of kidney function: A CKD prognosis consortium meta-analysis. European Heart Journal. 2018;**17**:1535-1542

[9] Lerma EV, Rosner M. Clinical Decisions in Nephrology and Hypertension and Kidney Transplantation. Chicago, USA: Springer; 2013

[10] Long B, Wanx JR, et al. Contraversies in management of hyperkalemia. Journal of Emergency Medicine. 2018;**55**(2):192-205

[11] Montford JR, Linas S. How dangerous is hyperkalemia? Journal of the American Society of Nephrology. 2017;**28**:3155-3165

[12] Mushiyakh Y, Danharia H, et al. Treatment and pathogenesis of acute hyperkalemia. Journal of Community Hospital Internal Medicine Perspectives. 2011;**1**:1-6

[13] Palmer BF. Regulation of potassium homeostasis, renal physiology. American Society of Nephrology. 2015;**10**:1050-1060

[14] Kovesdy CP. Potassium homeostasis in health and disease: A scientific workshop. American Journal of Kidney Diseases. 2017;**70**(6):844-858

[15] Pescribing Hypo-Electrolyte disturbances in Adults Protocol. Queensland Government. 2018

[16] Pescribing hyper-electrolyte disturbances in adults protocol. Queensland Government. 2018

[17] Rastegar A, Soleimani M. Electrolytes and acid-base disorders. NephSAP. 2017;**16**(1)

[18] Steddon S, Ashman N, Chesser A, et al. Oxford Handbook of Nephrology and Hypertension. UK: Oxford University Press; 2014

[19] Stern RH, Grief M, et al. Treatment of hyperkalemia: Something old and something new. Kidney International. 2016;**89**:546-554

[20] Viera AJ, Wouk N. Potassium disorders: Hypokalemia and hyperkalemia. American Family Physician. 2015;**92**(6):487-495

[21] Weaver CM, Stone MS, et al. What is the evidence base for a potassium requirement? Nutrition Today. 2018;**53**(5):184-195

[22] Weiner ID, Linas S, et al. Disorders of Potassium Metabolism, Comprehensive Clinical Nephrology. 6th ed. Elsevier; 2019. pp. 111-123